Aokigahara Forest: The Heartbreaking Secrets of Japan's Suicide Forest

Oliver Lancaster

Published by Oliver Lancaster, 2023.

AOKIGAHARA FOREST: THE HEARTBREAKING SECRETS OF JAPAN'S SUICIDE FOREST

First edition. July 15, 2023.

Copyright © 2023 Oliver Lancaster.

ISBN: 979-8223729358

Written by Oliver Lancaster.

Also by Oliver Lancaster

Chernobyl: Unveiling the tragedy. A Comprehensive Account of the Nuclear Disaster

The Bhopal Gas Tragedy: Unraveling the Catastrophe of 1984

The Deepwater Horizon Oil Spill of 2010: A Disaster Unveiled

Fukushima Fallout: Unveiling the Truth behind the 2011 Nuclear Disaster

Minamata Disease: Poisoned Waters and the Battle for Justice (1932-1968)

Evil Women: Unmasking History's Most Notorious Women

Bundy The Dark Chronicles: America's Infamous Serial Killer

Dahmer The Dark Chronicles: America's Infamous Milwaukee Cannibal

Zodiac The Dark Chronicles: America's Infamous Cryptic Killer

Bigfoot: The Comprehensive Investigation into the Elusive Legend

Chasing Legends: The Truth behind the Chupacabra

Chasing Legends: The Truth behind the Loch Ness Monster

Aokigahara Forest: The Heartbreaking Secrets of Japan's Suicide Forest

The Amityville House: The Haunting Secrets of America's Most Infamous Residence

The Tower of London: The Haunted Past and Secrets of Royal Ghosts
The Winchester Mystery House: The Riddle of Sarah Winchester's Mansion

Watch for more at https://tinyurl.com/olanc.

Sign up to my free newsletter to get updates on new releases, FREE teaser chapters to upcoming releases and FREE digital short stories.

Or visit https://tinyurl.com/olanc

I never spam and you can unsubscribe at any time.

OLIVER LANCASTER

Disclaimer

The information presented in this book, "Aokigahara Forest: The Heartbreaking Secrets of Japan's Suicide Forest," is based on extensive research and expert opinions. While every effort has been made to provide accurate and up-to-date information, readers are advised to consult professional sources and authorities for the most current data and advice regarding mental health, suicide prevention, and travel safety. The author and publisher shall not be held responsible for any actions or decisions made by readers based on the information contained within this book.

Aokigahara Forest: The Heartbreaking Secrets of Japan's Suicide Forest

OLIVER LANCASTER

Chapter 1: Introduction

Nestled at the northwest base of Mount Fuji, Aokigahara Forest stands as a place of both haunting beauty and profound sorrow. With its dense foliage, captivating natural features, and a reputation that has gained global recognition, this forest has captured the imaginations of many. However, its notoriety as the "Suicide Forest" has cast a dark shadow over its mystique.

Before delving into the forest's tragic reputation, it is important to appreciate the natural wonder of Aokigahara. With a name that translates to "Sea of Trees," the forest covers approximately 14 square miles (35 square kilometers) of land. Aokigahara is known for its thick growth of trees, moss-covered ground, and an eerily serene ambiance. The forest's unique geological history, shaped by volcanic activity, has created a landscape that is both captivating and foreboding.

Aokigahara Forest holds a special place in Japanese mythology and folklore. Legends speak of the forest as a mystical realm inhabited by supernatural creatures and the spirits of the departed. These tales have added to the allure and mystique surrounding Aokigahara, drawing in both curious adventurers and those seeking solace or answers in the depths of the forest.

Regrettably, Aokigahara Forest has gained international attention due to its association with suicide. The forest has been a site where individuals, facing deep despair and emotional anguish, have chosen to end their lives. The reason behind this unfortunate connection are complex an multifaceted, ranging from personal struggles to societa pressures. It is crucial to approach this subject matter wit empathy, recognizing the depth of human suffering involved.

To fully comprehend the significance of Aokigahara reputation, it is essential to explore the cultural context i which it has emerged. Japan has faced unique challenge related to mental health, societal expectations, and the stigm surrounding mental illness. These factors have contributed to higher suicide rate compared to many other developed nation Understanding the larger societal issues is essential in order t approach the topic of suicide in Aokigahara with sensitivit and respect.

Over the years, Aokigahara's reputation as the "Suicide Forest has been amplified by media coverage, both in Japan an internationally. Documentary films, news articles, an sensationalized portrayals have perpetuated the forest association with suicide, reinforcing its tragic image. Howeve it is important to acknowledge the role of responsibl journalism and media in raising awareness about mental healt issues and suicide prevention, encouraging importar conversations about support and understanding.

While the association of Aokigahara Forest with suicide undeniably heartbreaking, it is crucial to recognize that th reality is only one facet of the forest's story. Aokigahara ancient beauty, biodiversity, and cultural significance exten far beyond its tragic reputation. The forest holds a place i the hearts of many Japanese people who appreciate its natural splendor and value its historical and spiritual significance.

As we embark on this journey through the heartrending secrets of Aokigahara Forest, let us approach the subject matter with compassion and empathy. We will unravel the layers of history, delve into the societal issues that surround mental health and suicide, and explore the efforts being made to bring hope and healing to those affected. By doing so, we can shed light on the human experiences that have shaped this mystical forest and understand the importance of fostering a world where individuals find support and solace rather than despair within its depths.

Aokigahara Forest has long been intertwined with Japanese folklore and mythology, holding a deep cultural and historical significance. In ancient times, the forest was believed to be a gateway between the human world and the spirit realm. It was often depicted as a place where supernatural beings and spirits resided, creating an air of mystery and reverence around Aokigahara.

Shintoism, the indigenous religion of Japan, plays a significant role in shaping the cultural significance of Aokigahara Forest. Shinto beliefs emphasize the presence of kami, sacred spirits or deities, in natural elements such as mountains, rivers, and forests. Aokigahara, with its dense foliage, towering trees, and secluded atmosphere, was considered a sacred place, believed to be inhabited by powerful kami. The forest was regarded as a site for spiritual purification, meditation, and communion with nature.

Numerous legends and folklore have emerged around Aokigahara Forest, further enhancing its cultural significance. These tales often revolve around encounters with supernatural creatures, tragic love stories, and spirits of the departed. One popular legend tells the story of a yūrei, a vengeful ghost, who lures unsuspecting visitors deeper into the forest. These stories, passed down through generations, add to the mystique and allure of Aokigahara.

Aokigahara Forest has also inspired writers, poets, and artists throughout history. Its evocative atmosphere and rich symbolism have been depicted in various works of literature, poetry, and visual art. Japanese literary classics, such as "The Tale of Genji" by Murasaki Shikibu and the haiku of Matsuo Bashō, often make references to the forest's haunting beauty and spiritual significance. Artists have captured the forest's essence through paintings and woodblock prints, showcasing its serene yet melancholic allure.

In addition to its association with folklore, Aokigahara has served as a destination for pilgrimage throughout history. The forest's proximity to Mount Fuji, a sacred site in Japanese culture, has made it a part of religious journeys. Pilgrims would embark on treks to seek spiritual enlightenment, purification, and communion with nature. The forest's solitude and natural beauty provided a serene backdrop for introspection and contemplation.

Aokigahara Forest has witnessed significant historical events and cultural practices as well. During times of war, the forest provided a hiding place for soldiers and guerrilla fighters due to its dense vegetation and rugged terrain. The forest also served as a training ground for Buddhist monks, who sought seclusion and spiritual training amidst its tranquil surroundings.

While the forest's association with suicide has garnered attention in recent years, it is important to remember that Aokigahara's cultural significance extends beyond this tragic aspect. Many Japanese people still visit the forest for its spiritual ambiance, to connect with their cultural heritage, or to appreciate its natural beauty. Efforts are being made to preserve and protect the forest, promoting responsible tourism and fostering a deeper understanding of its cultural and historical significance.

Aokigahara Forest's cultural and historical significance in Japanese folklore is vast and multifaceted. Its portrayal in mythology, literature, art, and religious practices reflects the deep reverence and connection that the Japanese people have with nature and the spiritual realm. By understanding and appreciating the forest's cultural heritage, we can approach its tragic reputation with sensitivity and gain a more profound insight into the complexities of Aokigahara's story.

OLIVER LANCASTER

Chapter 2: Geographical Context

Aokigahara Forest, also known as the Sea of Trees, is situated in the northwest region of Honshu, the largest island of Japan. More specifically, it lies at the base of Mount Fuji, an iconic and sacred mountain in Japanese culture. The forest is part of the broader Fuji-Hakone-Izu National Park, which encompasses diverse natural landscapes, including volcanic peaks, lakes, and hot springs.

Aokigahara Forest covers an expansive area, spanning approximately 14 square miles (35 square kilometers) of land. Within its vast expanse, the forest boasts a captivating variety of flora and fauna, creating a rich and diverse ecosystem. The dense foliage, composed primarily of coniferous trees such as cedars and pines, contributes to the forest's distinct ambiance and otherworldly allure.

The unique geological features of Aokigahara Forest can be traced back to volcanic activity that occurred thousands of years ago. The forest is situated on a volcanic plateau formed by the lava flows from Mount Fuji's eruptions. Over time, the lava solidified into a basaltic rock known as Gotemba gravel, which serves as the foundation of the forest's soil. The porous nature of this gravel allows for excellent drainage, resulting in the growth of diverse plant life.

One of the remarkable characteristics of Aokigahara Forest is the extensive moss covering the forest floor. The moss thrives in the moist and shaded environment, creating a soft carpet of vibrant green. This dense layer of moss contributes to the forest's ethereal and mystical atmosphere, enhancing its allure and captivating visitors.

Aokigahara Forest is known for its intricate network of caves and ice caves, which add to its unique geological features. These caves were formed by ancient lava flows, creating natural tunnels and chambers beneath the forest's surface. Some of these caves contain ice formations that persist throughout the year due to the cool temperatures and volcanic activity in the area. These ice caves attract explorers and adventurers, providing a glimpse into the hidden depths of the forest.

Among the notable geological features within Aokigahara Forest is the Narusawa Ice Cave. Situated near the forest's edge, this cave offers a fascinating exploration opportunity. The cave's ice formations, shaped by freezing water drippings from the cave ceiling, create a surreal and mesmerizing sight. Visitors can wander through the icy corridors, admiring the natural beauty shaped by the interplay of fire and ice over time.

Adjacent to the Narusawa Ice Cave is another notable geological wonder, the Fugaku Wind Cave. This cave earned its name from the gusts of wind that flow through its passages. As visitors venture into the cave, they can feel the cool breeze generated by the temperature difference between the external air and the cave's interior. The Fugaku Wind Cave showcases the intricate balance of natural elements within Aokigahara Forest.

AOKIGAHARA FOREST: THE HEARTBREAKING SECRETS OF JAPAN'S SUICIDE FOREST

Aokigahara Forest's location at the base of Mount Fuji, its expansive size, and unique geological features make it a place of great fascination and wonder. The forest's origins in volcanic activity, the extensive moss covering the ground, and the presence of caves and ice formations all contribute to its captivating allure. Understanding the forest's geological context allows us to appreciate the intricate balance of natural forces that have shaped this mystical and enigmatic environment.

The proximity of Aokigahara Forest to Mount Fuji, one of Japan's most revered and iconic landmarks, adds to its significance and cultural value. Mount Fuji holds great spiritual and symbolic importance in Japanese culture, often regarded as a sacred site and a source of inspiration for artists, poets, and pilgrims. Aokigahara, nestled at the base of this majestic mountain, shares in the reverence and spiritual aura associated with Mount Fuji.

Aokigahara Forest's close relationship with Mount Fuji has provided inspiration for countless artists, writers, and poets throughout history. The serene and mystical atmosphere of the forest, combined with the majestic presence of Mount Fuji towering above, creates a compelling backdrop for creative expression. Many renowned works of art, literature, and poetry have drawn inspiration from the harmonious interplay between the forest and the mountain.

Aokigahara Forest's location within the Fuji-Hakone-Izu National Park further enhances its significance. This national park encompasses a diverse range of landscapes, including volcanic peaks, lakes, hot springs, and lush forests. The park's designation as a protected area ensures the preservation of its natural beauty and cultural heritage. Aokigahara Forest's inclusion within this national park emphasizes its importance as a valuable ecological and cultural asset.

The surrounding landscape, with its natural beauty and spiritual significance, has given rise to pilgrimage routes that traverse Aokigahara Forest. Pilgrims from various religious and spiritual traditions embark on these journeys, seeking enlightenment, purification, or a deeper connection with nature. The forest's tranquil ambiance and its association with Mount Fuji make it an integral part of these pilgrimage routes, providing a space for introspection and spiritual renewal.

The towering presence of Mount Fuji has a profound influence on the ecosystem within Aokigahara Forest. The mountain's volcanic activity, including its ash deposits and mineral-rich soils, contributes to the fertility of the surrounding lands. This, in turn, nurtures the diverse array of plant and animal life within the forest. The symbiotic relationship between Mount Fuji and Aokigahara Forest highlights the interconnectedness of the natural world.

The significance of Aokigahara's proximity to Mount Fuji and the surrounding landscape extends to conservation efforts and sustainable practices. Recognizing the forest's ecological importance, measures are in place to protect its biodiversity and maintain its natural integrity. Responsible tourism initiatives promote the appreciation of Aokigahara's beauty while minimizing the impact on its delicate ecosystem.

AOKIGAHARA FOREST: THE HEARTBREAKING SECRETS OF JAPAN'S SUICIDE FOREST

Conservation organizations work to raise awareness about the forest's fragility and advocate for its long-term preservation.

The combined allure of Aokigahara Forest and Mount Fuji has made the surrounding landscape a popular destination for tourists and nature enthusiasts. Visitors are drawn to the area's natural beauty, rich cultural heritage, and opportunities for outdoor activities. Cultural festivals, events, and guided tours celebrate the intertwined history of the forest, the mountain, and the surrounding landscape, offering visitors a chance to engage with the area's cultural and natural significance.

Aokigahara Forest's proximity to Mount Fuji and the surrounding landscape imbues it with profound significance. The spiritual and artistic inspiration derived from this close connection, the inclusion within the Fuji-Hakone-Izu National Park, and the presence of pilgrimage routes all underline the cultural and natural value of the forest. Recognizing and preserving this relationship ensures that future generations can continue to appreciate the harmonious interplay between Aokigahara Forest, Mount Fuji, and the captivating landscape that surrounds them.

OLIVER LANCASTER

Chapter 3: The Forest's Formation

Aokigahara Forest owes its geological formation to volcanic activity that occurred thousands of years ago. The forest lies on a volcanic plateau that was formed as a result of lava flows from Mount Fuji, an active stratovolcano. These volcanic eruptions played a pivotal role in shaping the landscape and geological features of the surrounding area, including the forest itself.

During eruptions, molten lava would flow from the volcanic vents and travel across the land, eventually reaching the area that is now Aokigahara Forest. As the lava cooled and solidified, it transformed into a type of basaltic rock known as Gotemba gravel. This basaltic rock forms the underlying foundation of the forest's soil composition and contributes to its unique geological characteristics.

The porous nature of the Gotemba gravel is crucial in shaping the soil composition within Aokigahara Forest. The permeable gravel allows for excellent drainage, preventing excessive water accumulation and creating a well-aerated environment for plant growth. This characteristic, combined with the abundant rainfall in the region, contributes to the flourishing vegetation and diverse flora found in the forest.

The presence of moss and fungi in Aokigahara Forest is another geological feature shaped by the unique soil composition. The porous nature of the Gotemba gravel allows for moisture retention, creating a damp and humid environment that is favorable for moss and fungi growth. As a result, the forest floor becomes adorned with vibrant moss coverings, creating a visually striking and otherworldly atmosphere.

Aokigahara Forest is also known for its extensive system of lava tube caves, which are formed by volcanic activity. Lava tube caves are created when the outer layer of a lava flow cools and solidifies while the molten lava inside continues to flow, eventually draining out and leaving behind a hollow tube-like structure. Over time, these lava tube caves form intricate networks beneath the forest surface, offering a unique geological feature for exploration.

In addition to lava tube caves, Aokigahara Forest is home to ice caves, further contributing to its geological diversity. These ice caves are formed when cold air from the surface flows into the lava tube caves, causing water to freeze and accumulate. The presence of ice formations within the caves creates an enchanting sight, adding to the ethereal ambiance of the forest.

While the initial formation of Aokigahara Forest can be attributed to volcanic activity, the geological processes shaping the forest continue to evolve over time. Erosion, weathering, and natural disturbances such as landslides and earthquakes play a role in altering the landscape. These ongoing geological processes contribute to the ever-changing nature of the forest, adding to its geological complexity and ecological resilience.

The geological formation of Aokigahara Forest is a testament to the powerful forces of volcanic activity that shaped the surrounding landscape. From the lava flows that created the basaltic rock foundation to the porous soil composition and the formation of lava tube caves and ice caves, the forest's unique geological features provide a glimpse into the Earth's dynamic processes. Understanding these geological processes helps us appreciate the intricate beauty and scientific significance of Aokigahara Forest.

Aokigahara Forest owes its distinct features and characteristics to the volcanic origins of the region. The forest is located in close proximity to Mount Fuji, an active stratovolcano, and the remnants of volcanic activity have shaped the landscape and contributed to the unique attributes of the forest.

Volcanic eruptions from Mount Fuji resulted in the outpouring of molten lava that flowed across the land, eventually reaching the area where Aokigahara Forest now stands. As the lava cooled and solidified, it transformed into a type of basaltic rock known as Gotemba gravel. The presence of this basaltic soil has had a significant influence on the forest's distinct features.

The basaltic soil of Aokigahara Forest is rich in minerals and nutrients derived from volcanic activity. As the lava disintegrated over time, it released these elements into the soil, creating a fertile environment for plant growth. The nutrient composition of the soil has played a crucial role in sustaining the diverse array of plant species that thrive in the forest.

The porous nature of the basaltic soil contributes to both moisture retention and efficient drainage within Aokigahara

Forest. The gravel composition allows the soil to retain moisture, creating a humid and damp environment that favors the growth of moss, fungi, and other moisture-loving vegetation. At the same time, the porous soil allows excess water to drain away, preventing waterlogging and maintaining suitable conditions for plant life.

The combination of the nutrient-rich basaltic soil, ample rainfall, and the forest's humid environment creates ideal conditions for the growth of moss. Aokigahara Forest is renowned for its extensive moss coverings, which create a visually striking carpet of vibrant green on the forest floor. The moss adds to the forest's otherworldly and mystical atmosphere, further enhancing its distinct features.

Volcanic activity played a crucial role in the formation of lava tube caves within Aokigahara Forest. As lava flowed during eruptions, the outer layer of the lava flow cooled and solidified, while the molten lava inside continued to flow. As the lava drained out, it left behind hollow tube-like structures known as lava tube caves. These geological formations are a unique and distinct feature of the forest, offering opportunities for exploration and adding to its allure.

The influence of volcanic activity on Aokigahara Forest has resulted in a diverse range of geological features and contributed to the forest's ecological resilience. From the nutrient-rich soil supporting diverse plant life to the presence of lava tube caves and the dynamic nature of the landscape, the forest exemplifies the intricate relationship between geological processes and the flourishing ecosystems they sustain.

AOKIGAHARA FOREST: THE HEARTBREAKING SECRETS OF JAPAN'S SUICIDE FOREST

Volcanic activity has left an indelible mark on Aokigahara Forest, shaping its distinct features and contributing to its natural allure. The lava flows, basaltic soil, moss-covered ground, lava tube caves, and other unique attributes of the forest are all manifestations of the influence of volcanic activity. Understanding the role of volcanism in shaping Aokigahara Forest provides insight into the dynamic processes that have sculpted this mystical environment and highlights the interconnectedness between geological forces and the vibrant ecosystems they support.

OLIVER LANCASTER

Chapter 4: Flora and Fauna

Aokigahara Forest is not only known for its haunting beauty and tragic reputation but also for its rich and diverse ecosystem. The forest is home to a wide array of plant and animal species, each playing a vital role in the delicate balance of this unique environment. Let us delve into the intricate web of life that thrives within the depths of Aokigahara.

Aokigahara Forest boasts a diverse range of flora, thanks to its fertile soil and favorable environmental conditions. The forest is primarily composed of coniferous trees, including Japanese cedar (Cryptomeria japonica), Japanese black pine (Pinus thunbergii), and Japanese hemlock (Tsuga sieboldii). These towering trees create a dense canopy that filters sunlight, creating a shaded and tranquil atmosphere beneath. The forest floor is adorned with a vibrant carpet of moss, ferns, and wildflowers, adding to the enchanting beauty of the landscape.

Within the forest, certain plant species have adapted to the specific conditions of Aokigahara. The Ranzania japonica, or the Fuji blue daylily, is a rare and endangered flower that blooms in the area surrounding Mount Fuji. It displays striking blue-violet petals and serves as a symbol of the forest's resilience and natural beauty. A variety of lichens and fungi also thrive in the damp and shaded environment, contributing to the forest's ecological diversity.

Aokigahara Forest provides a habitat for numerous bird species, both resident and migratory. The forest's dense foliage and abundance of insects attract a variety of avian visitors. Species such as the varied tit (Poecile varius), Japanese bush warbler (Cettia diphone), and great spotted woodpecker (Dendrocopos major) can be spotted among the branches. These birds contribute to the forest's soundscape with their melodic songs, adding to its serene and natural ambiance.

Aokigahara Forest is inhabited by a diverse range of mammals and small creatures. Sika deer (Cervus nippon) can be seen grazing among the trees, while Asian black bears (Ursus thibetanus) occasionally roam the forest in search of food. Other mammals, including foxes (Vulpes vulpes), wild boar (Sus scrofa), and Japanese martens (Martes melampus), are also found in the area. Additionally, the forest is home to a variety of small creatures, such as rabbits, rodents, and numerous insect species, all playing essential roles in the forest ecosystem.

The moist and shaded environment of Aokigahara Forest supports a diverse population of amphibians and reptiles. Japanese giant salamanders (Andrias japonicus), endemic to Japan, can be found in the forest's streams and waterways. Various frog species, such as the Japanese tree frog (Hyla japonica) and the Japanese brown frog (Rana japonica), also thrive within the forest's ecosystems. Reptiles such as the Japanese rat snake (Elaphe climacophora) and the Japanese grass lizard (Takydromus tachydromoides) can be found basking in patches of sunlight.

AOKIGAHARA FOREST: THE HEARTBREAKING SECRETS OF JAPAN'S SUICIDE FOREST

The interconnectedness of the diverse species within Aokigahara Forest creates a delicate ecological balance. The plants provide food and shelter for the animals, while the animals contribute to seed dispersal and pollination. The decomposition of organic matter by insects and microorganisms enriches the soil, nurturing plant growth. This intricate web of interactions ensures the sustainability and resilience of the forest ecosystem.

Aokigahara Forest is not only a place of tragic history and haunting beauty but also a thriving ecosystem. The diversity of flora and fauna within the forest highlights the resilience and adaptability of life in even the harshest of environments. Understanding and appreciating the intricate relationships between the various species within Aokigahara contributes to the importance of preserving and protecting this unique and precious ecosystem for future generations to appreciate and learn from.

Aokigahara Forest is home to a diverse array of plant and animal species, some of which are unique to this particular environment. These species have adapted to the forest's specific conditions, contributing to its ecological richness and distinctiveness. Let us explore some of the notable plant and animal species that thrive within the depths of Aokigahara.

Ranzania japonica (Fuji Blue Daylily): This rare and endangered flower is a symbol of the resilience and beauty of Aokigahara Forest. The Fuji Blue Daylily displays stunning blue-violet petals and blooms in the area surrounding Mount Fuji.

Pteridium aquilinum (Bracken Fern): Bracken ferns are abundant in Aokigahara Forest and contribute to its lush undergrowth. These ferns have large fronds and adapt well to the shaded and moist environment of the forest.

Epipogium roseum (Ghost Orchid): The ghost orchid is a rare and elusive orchid species found in the forest. It is known for its delicate, pale pink flowers that seem to emerge mysteriously from the forest floor.

Sasa kurilensis (Kuril Bamboo): This species of bamboo is found in Aokigahara Forest and creates dense thickets that provide cover and habitat for various animals. The bamboo's sturdy stems and broad leaves add to the forest's enchanting ambiance.

Nucifraga caryocatactes (Eurasian Nutcracker): The Eurasian nutcracker is a bird species commonly found in Aokigahara Forest. These birds play a vital role in seed dispersal, as they have a fondness for collecting and caching nuts and seeds for future consumption.

Emberiza cioides (Meadow Bunting): The meadow bunting is a small bird species that thrives in the forest's grassy clearings and open spaces. Its melodious song adds to the tranquil atmosphere of the forest.

Parus varius (Varied Tit): The varied tit is a colorful bird species with a distinctive pattern of black, white, and yellow feathers. These small birds can be seen flitting among the trees, foraging for insects and seeds.

AOKIGAHARA FOREST: THE HEARTBREAKING SECRETS OF JAPAN'S SUICIDE FOREST

Cervus nippon (Sika Deer): Sika deer roam the forest, adding grace and beauty to the landscape. These herbivorous mammals play an essential role in shaping the vegetation of Aokigahara through their browsing and grazing habits.

Ursus thibetanus (Asian Black Bear): Though rarely encountered, Asian black bears occasionally inhabit the forest. They are an iconic species of the region and contribute to the forest's biodiversity and ecological balance.

Martes melampus (Japanese Marten): The Japanese marten is a small carnivorous mammal found in Aokigahara Forest. These agile hunters help control populations of small rodents and insects, maintaining the balance of the forest's ecosystem.

Andrias japonicus (Japanese Giant Salamander): The Japanese giant salamander is a fascinating and rare amphibian species found in the forest's streams and waterways. These large, aquatic creatures are the largest known salamanders in the world.

Takydromus tachydromoides (Japanese Grass Lizard): The Japanese grass lizard is a reptile species that inhabits the forest floor and grassy areas. These agile lizards are known for their vibrant green coloration and darting movements.

Hyla japonica (Japanese Tree Frog): The Japanese tree frog is a common amphibian species in Aokigahara Forest. Their distinctive calls can be heard during the summer months, adding to the forest's natural soundtrack.

The unique plant and animal species within Aokigahara Forest contribute to the overall ecological significance of the area. Each species plays a specific role in the forest's food web, nutrient cycling, pollination, and seed dispersal. The interdependence of these species helps maintain the delicate balance and resilience of the forest's ecosystem.

Aokigahara Forest is teeming with unique and fascinating plant and animal species that have adapted to the specific conditions of this mystical environment. From the rare Fuji Blue Daylily and ghost orchid to the diverse bird, mammal, reptile, and amphibian species, each contributes to the intricate web of life within the forest. Recognizing the importance of these species highlights the need for conservation efforts to protect the biodiversity and natural heritage of Aokigahara for future generations to appreciate and study.

AOKIGAHARA FOREST: THE HEARTBREAKING SECRETS OF JAPAN'S SUICIDE FOREST

Chapter 5: Mythology and Legends

Aokigahara Forest, with its enigmatic ambiance and haunting reputation, has become the subject of numerous folklore and mythical stories. These tales have contributed to the forest's mystique and captivated the imaginations of people for centuries. Let us delve into the folklore and mythical narratives associated with Aokigahara.

In Japanese folklore, Aokigahara Forest is often depicted as a realm inhabited by yūrei, the spirits of the departed. According to these stories, those who died tragically or took their own lives within the forest become restless spirits trapped in its depths. Legends describe these yūrei as vengeful or sorrowful entities that seek to lure unsuspecting visitors further into the forest. These tales have fostered beliefs in the supernatural and contributed to the forest's reputation as a place of eerie encounters.

The presence of yūrei in Aokigahara Forest is deeply intertwined with Japanese folklore and cultural beliefs. In traditional folklore, yūrei are believed to be spirits unable to find peace due to unresolved emotional issues or untimely deaths. Their restless spirits are said to roam specific locations, such as Aokigahara, seeking resolution or release from their tormented existence. The forest, with its dense vegetation and secluded atmosphere, has become a significant setting for these yūrei narratives.

One of the most well-known folktales associated with Aokigahara Forest is the story of the Okiko doll. According to the legend, a young girl named Okiko owned a cherished doll. When Okiko tragically died, her spirit became attached to the doll. It is said that visitors to the forest may come across the Okiko doll, which is believed to be possessed by the girl's spirit. The doll is said to move on its own and emit ghostly cries, perpetuating the eerie reputation of the forest.

Aokigahara Forest is also believed to be inhabited by various supernatural creatures in Japanese folklore. Folktales speak of encounters with kappa, mischievous water-dwelling creatures, who are said to be drawn to the forest's streams and waterways. Other stories mention tengu, legendary creatures with avian features, who are believed to reside within the forest's dense foliage. These supernatural beings add to the sense of mystery and wonder surrounding Aokigahara.

Certain areas within Aokigahara Forest are believed to be cursed or imbued with negative energy. Folklore warns against entering these forbidden grounds, as they are said to bring misfortune or invite the wrath of vengeful spirits. These areas may be marked by eerie silence, unusual rock formations, or twisted trees, heightening the sense of foreboding and caution associated with the forest.

The folklore and mythical stories surrounding Aokigahara Forest hold cultural significance and convey important lessons. They often highlight the consequences of despair, the importance of resolving emotional turmoil, and the consequences of intruding upon sacred or forbidden spaces.

These tales serve as cautionary reminders and encourage respect for the spiritual and natural realms.

The folklore and mythical stories associated with Aokigahara Forest add layers of intrigue and mystique to its already haunting reputation. Tales of yūrei, encounters with supernatural beings, and the warnings of cursed areas contribute to the forest's cultural significance and provide insights into Japanese folklore and beliefs. By exploring these narratives, we can gain a deeper understanding of the forest's cultural heritage and the lessons embedded within these tales.

The legends and folklore surrounding Aokigahara Forest have had a profound influence on local beliefs and cultural practices. These stories, passed down through generations, have shaped the perception of the forest and contributed to the development of traditions, rituals, and beliefs among the local communities. Let us explore the impact of these legends on the beliefs and practices associated with Aokigahara Forest.

The legends of yūrei and supernatural beings inhabiting Aokigahara Forest have fostered a deep sense of spirituality and reverence for nature among the local communities. The forest is seen as a sacred place where the spiritual and natural realms intertwine. Visitors and locals alike may approach the forest with a sense of respect and caution, recognizing the potential presence of otherworldly forces and the need to maintain harmony with the environment.

In response to the legends and beliefs associated with Aokigahara Forest, certain rituals and offerings have emerged as cultural practices. Some individuals and religious groups may perform rituals or prayers to honor and appease the spirits believed to reside within the forest. Offerings of flowers, incense, and other symbolic items are often made at designated spots or sacred areas as a sign of respect and reverence.

The legends of Aokigahara Forest have also contributed to the tradition of pilgrimages and spiritual journeys to the area. For some, the forest represents a place of introspection, spiritual purification, or seeking enlightenment. People embark on treks to Aokigahara, often in conjunction with visits to Mount Fuji, to connect with nature, engage in self-reflection, and deepen their spiritual practices.

The legends surrounding Aokigahara Forest serve as cautionary tales, reminding people of the consequences of despair, the importance of mental well-being, and the need for respect when entering sacred spaces. These stories provide valuable lessons and reinforce cultural values related to empathy, compassion, and the preservation of one's mental and emotional health. They encourage individuals to approach the forest with sensitivity and care.

The tragic reputation of Aokigahara Forest has sparked awareness about mental health issues and suicide prevention. Recognizing the vulnerability of those who may be struggling emotionally, local communities, government organizations, and support groups have taken steps to raise awareness, provide resources, and offer counseling services. Efforts have been made to shift the narrative surrounding the forest by focusing on mental health education and support rather than solely perpetuating the legends associated with suicide.

The legends and cultural significance of Aokigahara Forest have contributed to the recognition of the forest's ecological value and the need for its conservation. The forest's association with spiritual practices and its status as a symbol of natural beauty have motivated efforts to preserve its biodiversity, protect its unique ecosystem, and promote sustainable tourism practices. Environmental awareness and education initiatives emphasize the importance of respecting and preserving the forest for future generations.

The legends and folklore surrounding Aokigahara Forest have left a lasting impact on local beliefs and cultural practices. These stories have instilled a sense of spirituality, reverence for nature, and caution among the local communities. The legends serve as cautionary tales and remind individuals of the importance of mental well-being and the need for empathy and compassion. Furthermore, the legends have spurred awareness about mental health issues and environmental conservation efforts. By acknowledging and respecting the influence of these legends, communities can preserve the cultural heritage associated with Aokigahara Forest while promoting understanding, compassion, and sustainability.

OLIVER LANCASTER

Chapter 6: Historical Significance

AOKIGAHARA FOREST HAS a rich historical background that predates its reputation as the "Suicide Forest." The forest holds cultural significance, as it has been associated with Japanese folklore, spiritual practices, and artistic inspiration for centuries. The serene beauty and mystical ambiance of the forest have captivated people throughout history.

The reputation of Aokigahara Forest as the "Suicide Forest" emerged in the 1960s, influenced by various factors. Japan was experiencing a period of social and economic change, leading to increased social pressures and mental health challenges. The forest's seclusion, dense vegetation, and tragic history began to attract individuals contemplating suicide, leading to a rise in suicide rates within the forest.

The reputation of Aokigahara Forest as a suicide hotspot gained further traction through media coverage and its portrayal in popular culture. Documentaries, news reports, and literary works shed light on the forest's tragic reputation, attracting international attention. Aokigahara became a subject of fascination for filmmakers, authors, and artists, further perpetuating its dark image in popular culture.

Recognizing the challenges associated with suicide rates in Aokigahara Forest, the Japanese government implemented various initiatives to address the issue. Warning signs were placed at the forest's entrances, encouraging individuals to seek help and think about their families. The goal was to discourage suicide attempts and raise awareness about mental health resources available to those in need.

In response to the forest's reputation, numerous volunteer groups and organizations emerged to patrol and monitor the forest, aiming to prevent suicide attempts and provide support to individuals in distress. These groups work tirelessly to raise awareness about mental health, provide emotional support, and promote suicide prevention initiatives in the surrounding communities.

In recent years, there has been a shift in the narrative surrounding Aokigahara Forest. Efforts have focused on promoting mental health awareness, encouraging open dialogue about mental well-being, and providing resources and support to individuals in crisis. Mental health organizations and counseling services have become more prominent, aiming to address the underlying issues leading to suicides in the forest.

Aokigahara Forest's reputation has also prompted efforts to balance environmental conservation and responsible tourism practices. The delicate ecosystem of the forest requires protection, and initiatives have been implemented to promote sustainable tourism, minimize the impact of visitors, and raise awareness about the importance of preserving the forest's natural beauty and biodiversity.

AOKIGAHARA FOREST: THE HEARTBREAKING SECRETS OF JAPAN'S SUICIDE FOREST

Aokigahara Forest's reputation as the "Suicide Forest" has evolved over time, influenced by historical events and milestones. From its cultural significance and early associations with folklore to its tragic reputation and subsequent media coverage, the forest has faced significant challenges. However, there has been a recent shift towards promoting mental health awareness, suicide prevention, and environmental conservation. By acknowledging the historical events and milestones that have shaped its reputation, communities can work towards changing the narrative surrounding Aokigahara Forest and fostering a more compassionate and sustainable future.

Aokigahara Forest, known for its haunting beauty and tragic reputation, also played a significant role during World War II. The forest served as a vital resource for the local community and was intimately connected to the war effort. This chapter explores the forest's role during this tumultuous period and its impact on the local community.

During World War II, Japan faced a severe shortage of resources, including timber, which was essential for various military needs. Aokigahara Forest, with its dense vegetation and vast expanse, became a valuable source of timber for the production of weapons, construction materials, and fuel. Local residents were enlisted to harvest trees from the forest, contributing to the war effort.

The local community surrounding Aokigahara Forest faced the impact of wartime policies, including forced labor. Residents were often conscripted to work in logging operations within the forest, where they felled trees and assisted in processing timber. The labor conditions were demanding, and the community had to endure physical hardships and emotional strain during this challenging period.

The intensive logging operations in Aokigahara Forest during World War II had a significant environmental impact. The removal of large numbers of trees disrupted the forest ecosystem, causing disturbances to wildlife habitats and altering the natural balance. The consequences of these actions on the forest's biodiversity and long-term sustainability were felt for years to come.

The war had broader socioeconomic effects on the local community surrounding Aokigahara Forest. The forced labor and redirection of resources towards the war effort resulted in shifts in the community's livelihoods and economic activities. Traditional occupations, such as farming and forestry, were temporarily displaced as the focus shifted to meeting wartime demands.

The impact of World War II on the local community and Aokigahara Forest left enduring memories and shaped the collective resilience of the people. The hardships faced during the war fostered a sense of unity and determination among the community members. The memories of those challenging times have been passed down through generations, serving as a reminder of the resilience and strength of the local community.

After the war, the local community and the forest underwent a period of recovery. Efforts were made to restore the forest ecosystem and protect its natural beauty. Conservation initiatives were implemented to mitigate the environmental impact of logging and ensure the long-term sustainability of Aokigahara Forest.

Aokigahara Forest played a significant role during World War I, serving as a valuable resource for timber and contributing to the war effort. The local community endured the hardships of forced labor and witnessed the environmental impact of intensive logging operations. However, the community's resilience and enduring memories of that time have shaped their collective identity. Post-war recovery efforts focused on conservation and sustainability, recognizing the importance of preserving the forest's natural beauty and protecting its delicate ecosystem. Understanding the forest's role during World War I provides insights into the historical context and its lasting impact on both the environment and the local community.

Chapter 7: A Dark Reputation

Aokigahara Forest, nestled at the base of Mount Fuji, has gained global recognition as a suicide hotspot. The rise of Aokigahara as a site for suicide is a complex phenomenon influenced by various factors. This chapter examines the underlying causes and contributing factors that have led to the forest's unfortunate reputation.

Stigma and Shame: In Japanese society, mental health issues and suicide have historically carried a stigma, often resulting in individuals feeling ashamed and isolated. This stigma may prevent individuals from seeking help and lead them to consider secluded locations such as Aokigahara Forest.

Social Pressure: Japan's cultural emphasis on conformity and social expectations can exert immense pressure on individuals, particularly during times of economic hardship or personal challenges. The burden of meeting societal expectations and the fear of failure can contribute to feelings of despair and hopelessness.

Media Influence: The media's coverage of suicides in Aokigahara Forest has played a significant role in perpetuating its reputation as a suicide hotspot. Sensationalized reporting and graphic imagery can contribute to copycat behavior and romanticized notions of suicide among vulnerable individuals.

Seclusion and Privacy: Aokigahara Forest's dense vegetation and remote location provide a secluded and private setting for individuals contemplating suicide. The forest's vastness can make it difficult for rescue efforts and contributes to the sense of anonymity for those seeking to end their lives.

Dark and Eerie Atmosphere: The haunting beauty and eerie ambiance of Aokigahara Forest may resonate with individuals experiencing deep emotional distress. The forest's reputation, intertwined with legends of yūrei and tragic folklore, adds to its allure as a place of escape.

Symbolism and Finality: Aokigahara Forest's association with death and its history of suicides may make it appear as a symbolic location for individuals seeking a definitive end to their suffering. The symbolism attached to the forest can create a sense of attraction for those contemplating suicide.

Mental Health Awareness: Historically, mental health issues and suicide prevention have not received sufficient attention and support in Japan. Limited access to mental health services and the stigma associated with seeking help can contribute to individuals feeling isolated and hopeless.

Support Systems: Inadequate support systems and a lack of accessible mental health resources in the surrounding areas may contribute to individuals feeling helpless and without the necessary support to address their emotional distress.

Signage and Patrols: The placement of warning signs at the entrances of Aokigahara Forest aims to deter individuals from attempting suicide and encourage them to seek help. Volunteer patrols and increased surveillance have also been implemented to identify and provide support to individuals in distress.

Mental Health Initiatives: There has been a growing recognition of the importance of mental health education and awareness in Japan. Efforts to promote mental health initiatives, provide counseling services, and reduce the stigma surrounding mental health are gradually gaining momentum.

Suicide Prevention Organizations: Various organizations and support groups are actively involved in suicide prevention efforts, focusing on raising awareness, providing helplines, and offering community-based resources to those in need.

The rise of Aokigahara Forest as a suicide hotspot is a complex phenomenon influenced by a combination of sociocultural, geographical, psychological, and systemic factors. The stigma surrounding mental health, societal pressures, media influence, and the forest's unique characteristics all contribute to its unfortunate reputation. Efforts focused on mental health awareness, support systems, and suicide prevention initiatives are crucial in addressing the underlying issues and providing individuals with the help they need. By understanding the multifaceted nature of the problem, it becomes possible to develop comprehensive strategies to prevent suicide and promote mental well-being within the community.

The phenomenon of Aokigahara Forest as a suicide hotspot is influenced by a complex interplay of social and psychological factors. This chapter delves into the underlying social and psychological dynamics that contribute to the prevalence of suicide in the forest.

Stigma and Shame: In Japanese society, mental health issues and suicide have long carried a strong stigma. Individuals experiencing emotional distress may feel ashamed and reluctant to seek help due to fear of judgment and social exclusion. The stigma surrounding mental health can hinder open discussions and prevent individuals from accessing necessary support.

Cultural Pressure and Expectations: Japan's societal norms place a significant emphasis on conformity and meeting social expectations. The pressure to succeed academically, professionally, and socially can be overwhelming. Individuals who struggle to meet these expectations may feel immense shame and perceive suicide as a way out of their perceived failures.

Isolation and Loneliness: Modern lifestyles and societal changes have contributed to increased feelings of isolation and loneliness among individuals. Factors such as urbanization, changing family structures, and a focus on individualism can create a sense of disconnection from supportive social networks. This isolation can exacerbate feelings of despair and hopelessness.

Mental Health Disorders: Underlying mental health disorders, such as depression, anxiety, and mood disorders, play a significant role in suicide. Individuals with untreated or undiagnosed mental health conditions may experience persistent feelings of sadness, despair, and hopelessness, making them more susceptible to suicidal ideation.

Desperation and Psychological Pain: Intense emotional pain, coupled with a perceived lack of viable alternatives, can lead individuals to consider suicide as a means to escape their suffering. The forest's seclusion and reputation for offering solitude may appeal to individuals seeking a place to carry out their final act.

Copycat Behavior: The phenomenon of suicide contagion, or copycat behavior, can contribute to the clustering of suicides in specific locations. Media coverage and sensationalized portrayals of suicides in Aokigahara Forest may inadvertently create a sense of romanticism or fascination with the act, leading vulnerable individuals to view the forest as a desirable destination for ending their lives.

Limited Mental Health Resources: Access to mental health services and support can be limited, especially in rural areas where Aokigahara Forest is located. Sparse availability of mental health professionals and long waiting times for treatment can create barriers to timely help-seeking.

Lack of Awareness and Education: Limited awareness and understanding of mental health issues may prevent individuals from recognizing their own struggles or seeking help for themselves or others. Education and awareness campaigns that destigmatize mental health and promote help-seeking behaviors are essential in addressing this barrier.

Mental Health Promotion: Initiatives aimed at promotin mental health awareness, emotional well-being, and resilienc are crucial in combating the underlying factors contributin to suicide. Promoting a culture of openness, empathy, an understanding can help reduce stigma and encourage earl intervention.

Enhanced Mental Health Services: Expanding access t mental health services, particularly in rural areas, is vital fo individuals seeking support. Increasing the number of ment health professionals, improving community-based services, an implementing crisis helplines can help address help-seekin barriers.

Responsible Media Reporting: Media organizations play significant role in shaping public perceptions of suicid Promoting responsible reporting guidelines that emphasiz empathy, avoid sensationalism, and provide appropriat resources for help can contribute to reducing the risk of suicid contagion.

The prevalence of suicide in Aokigahara Forest is influenced b a complex interplay of social and psychological factors. Stigm cultural pressures, isolation, mental health disorders, an help-seeking barriers all contribute to this phenomenon. T address the issue, comprehensive prevention strategies shoul focus on reducing stigma, increasing awareness, improvin mental health resources, and fostering supportiv environments. By addressing the underlying social an psychological factors, it becomes possible to create a societ that promotes mental well-being and supports individuals in crisis.

Chapter 8: Cultural Perspectives

Understanding the Japanese perception of suicide and the stigmas surrounding mental health is crucial for comprehending the context in which Aokigahara Forest's suicide phenomenon occurs. This chapter examines the cultural and societal factors that shape the Japanese perception of suicide and contribute to the stigmatization of mental health.

Historical Attitudes: Throughout Japanese history, suicide has been viewed through various lenses, including notions of honor, shame, and sacrifice. Practices such as seppuku (ritual suicide) were once prevalent, highlighting the cultural complexities surrounding suicide.

Influences of Buddhism: Buddhism, a dominant religion in Japan, traditionally views suicide as an act with negative consequences, as it disrupts the natural order of life and carries karmic implications. However, Buddhist beliefs also emphasize compassion and understanding, which can be instrumental in promoting mental well-being.

Collectivism and Social Harmony: Japanese society places great emphasis on collectivism and maintaining social harmony. This collective mindset can discourage individuals from openly discussing their personal struggles or seeking help for fear of burdening others or disrupting social cohesion.

Concept of "Honne" and "Tatemae": The cultural concept of honne (true feelings) and tatemae (public face) can contribute to a lack of open dialogue about mental health. Individuals may feel compelled to present a facade of emotional well-being, even when they are struggling internally, reinforcing the stigma associated with admitting vulnerabilities.

Perceived Burden: Individuals in Japan may hesitate to seek help for mental health issues due to the fear of burdening their families or the broader community. The desire to protect loved ones from emotional distress can prevent open discussions and hinder access to necessary support.

Shame and Social Consequences: Mental health struggles are often accompanied by feelings of shame and guilt in Japanese society. The stigma associated with mental health issues can lead individuals to hide their struggles, preventing them from seeking help and perpetuating the cycle of silence and shame.

Professional Consequences: Disclosing mental health issues in the workplace can carry negative implications, including potential discrimination and career setbacks. The fear of professional repercussions further discourages individuals from seeking support or discussing their challenges openly.

Lack of Understanding: Limited awareness and understanding of mental health issues contribute to the stigmatization of mental health in Japan. Misconceptions and stereotypes surrounding mental illness can foster fear and prejudice, hindering empathy and supportive attitudes.

AOKIGAHARA FOREST: THE HEARTBREAKING SECRETS OF JAPAN'S SUICIDE FOREST

Rising Mental Health Awareness: In recent years, Japan has witnessed a shift in attitudes toward mental health. Greater public awareness campaigns, educational initiatives, and personal stories shared by individuals have helped reduce stigma and increase understanding.

Improved Mental Health Services: Efforts have been made to expand mental health services and resources in Japan. Increased accessibility to mental health professionals, counseling services, and helplines has been instrumental in providing support for those in need.

Advocacy and Support Groups: Various organizations and advocacy groups are actively working to promote mental health awareness, provide resources, and reduce stigma. These initiatives aim to create a supportive environment and foster empathy and understanding surrounding mental health.

The perception of suicide in Japan and the stigmas surrounding mental health are deeply rooted in cultural and societal factors. The cultural emphasis on collectivism, the concepts of honne and tatemae, and the fear of shame and burden contribute to the stigmatization of mental health struggles. However, changing perspectives and increased mental health awareness initiatives are gradually challenging these stigmas. By fostering open dialogue, promoting empathy, and providing accessible support systems, Japan can continue to make progress in addressing mental health issues and reducing the associated stigmas.

Aokigahara Forest's reputation as the "Suicide Forest" is influenced by various cultural and societal aspects. This chapter examines the intersections between these factors and the forest's reputation, shedding light on the complex dynamics at play.

Folklore and Legends: Aokigahara Forest's association with yūrei (spirits of the departed) and supernatural beings in Japanese folklore contributes to its mystique and haunting reputation. These legends have shaped the cultural perception of the forest as a place of spiritual significance and otherworldly encounters.

Spiritual Practices: The forest's serene and secluded atmosphere has attracted spiritual practitioners and seekers throughout history. Some individuals view Aokigahara as a place for introspection, purification, and spiritual experiences, intertwining the forest with spiritual beliefs and practices.

Artistic Inspiration: Aokigahara Forest has served as a muse for artists, writers, and poets who have been drawn to its ethereal beauty and melancholic allure. Paintings, literature, and poems inspired by the forest have contributed to its cultural significance and its representation in artistic works.

Literary Works: The forest's tragic reputation and folklore have been explored in Japanese literature. Novels, short stories, and poems have delved into the psychological and emotional depths associated with Aokigahara, capturing the complex intersection between the forest's reputation and the human experience.

AOKIGAHARA FOREST: THE HEARTBREAKING SECRETS OF JAPAN'S SUICIDE FOREST

Media Coverage: The forest's reputation as a suicide hotspot has received extensive media coverage, both within Japan and internationally. Documentaries, news reports, and online content have contributed to the dissemination of its tragic image, perpetuating its notoriety.

Pop Culture References: Aokigahara Forest has been referenced in various forms of popular culture, including films, music, and literature beyond Japan's borders. These references often emphasize the forest's eerie reputation and its association with tragedy, further embedding its image in the collective consciousness.

Shifting Mental Health Perspectives: The rise of mental health awareness and the recognition of the importance of suicide prevention have intersected with Aokigahara Forest's reputation. Efforts to address mental health issues and reduce stigma have prompted discussions about the underlying causes of suicide and the need for support systems.

Support Organizations: Numerous organizations and volunteer groups are dedicated to suicide prevention and supporting individuals in crisis. These initiatives intersect with the forest's reputation by actively patrolling the area, raising awareness, and providing helplines and resources to those in need.

Dark Tourism: Aokigahara Forest has become a destination for dark tourism, attracting visitors intrigued by its tragic reputation. This intersection of tourism and tragedy raises ethical considerations, as responsible tourism practices should prioritize sensitivity, respect for the local community, and the preservation of the forest's natural environment.

Conservation Efforts: The forest's reputation has prompted conservation initiatives aimed at protecting its unique ecosystem and preserving its natural beauty. Balancing the preservation of Aokigahara with the influx of visitors requires careful management and environmental awareness.

The reputation of Aokigahara Forest intersects with various cultural and societal aspects, influencing its perception and global recognition. Folklore, spirituality, artistic inspiration, media portrayal, mental health awareness, and tourism all contribute to the complex dynamics surrounding the forest's reputation. Recognizing these intersections allows for a more nuanced understanding of the cultural and societal factors at play, facilitating discussions on mental health, conservation, and responsible engagement with the forest.

AOKIGAHARA FOREST: THE HEARTBREAKING SECRETS OF JAPAN'S SUICIDE FOREST

Chapter 9: Conservation Efforts

Recognizing the ecological significance and unique biodiversity of Aokigahara Forest, various conservation initiatives have been implemented to preserve and protect this natural treasure. This chapter explores the conservation efforts dedicated to safeguarding the forest's delicate ecosystem and promoting sustainable practices.

Public Outreach and Education: Conservation organizations and local authorities have undertaken initiatives to raise awareness about Aokigahara Forest's environmental importance. Educational programs, guided tours, and informational campaigns are conducted to foster an understanding of the forest's ecological significance and the need for its preservation.

Environmental Impact Assessments: Comprehensive assessments of the forest's environmental impact have been conducted to evaluate the potential consequences of human activities and guide conservation efforts. These assessments provide valuable data to inform sustainable management strategies and protect the forest's fragile ecosystem.

Responsible Tourism Practices: In response to the growing interest in Aokigahara Forest as a tourist destination, efforts have been made to promote responsible tourism practices. Guidelines and regulations aim to minimize the impact of visitors on the environment, preserve the forest's integrity, and promote respectful behavior.

Guided Tours and Interpretive Centers: Local authorities and conservation organizations have established guided tours and interpretive centers to offer visitors an educational experience that highlights the forest's natural features, ecological importance, and conservation efforts. These initiatives help foster a deeper understanding and appreciation for the forest while ensuring responsible visitation.

Reforestation Programs: To mitigate the impact of historical logging activities and maintain the forest's biodiversity, reforestation programs have been implemented. These initiatives involve planting native tree species and promoting natural regeneration, aiding in the restoration of the forest's ecological balance.

Invasive Species Management: Invasive plant species can disrupt the forest ecosystem and threaten the survival of native flora and fauna. Conservation initiatives focus on the removal and control of invasive species, allowing the native vegetation to thrive and supporting the recovery of the forest's natural habitats.

Biodiversity Studies: Ongoing research and monitoring programs help assess and document the forest's biodiversity. These studies provide valuable insights into the flora, fauna, and ecological processes within Aokigahara, facilitating informed conservation strategies and ensuring the long-term health of the forest.

AOKIGAHARA FOREST: THE HEARTBREAKING SECRETS OF JAPAN'S SUICIDE FOREST

Wildlife Protection: Conservation efforts extend to the protection of wildlife within Aokigahara Forest. Monitoring programs and measures to safeguard endangered species, such as the Asian black bear and numerous bird species, contribute to the preservation of the forest's ecological balance.

Government and Local Authorities: The Japanese government and local authorities play a crucial role in coordinating conservation efforts and implementing regulations to protect Aokigahara Forest. They work in collaboration with conservation organizations, researchers, and local communities to ensure the effective management and preservation of the forest.

Community Engagement: Engaging local communities is vital for the success of conservation initiatives. Involving residents in decision-making processes, supporting sustainable livelihoods, and raising awareness about the importance of preserving Aokigahara foster a sense of ownership and stewardship among the local community.

Conservation initiatives for Aokigahara Forest reflect a collective commitment to preserving its ecological integrity and promoting sustainable practices. Through environmental awareness, responsible tourism, reforestation programs, invasive species management, research, and collaborative partnerships, dedicated efforts are made to protect the forest's delicate ecosystem. By implementing these conservation measures, Aokigahara Forest can continue to thrive as a natural treasure, providing valuable habitats for wildlife and offering a serene and biodiverse environment for future generations to appreciate and enjoy.

Preserving the ecological balance of Aokigahara Forest while addressing its dark history poses unique challenges. This chapter examines the complexities and difficulties faced in maintaining the forest's delicate ecosystem while acknowledging its tragic reputation and the associated mental health issues.

Balancing Conservation and Awareness: Striking a balance between conservation efforts and raising awareness about mental health is essential. While it is crucial to protect the forest's biodiversity, it is equally important to approach the forest's dark history with sensitivity, respect, and compassion.

Minimizing Environmental Impact: Conservation initiatives must prioritize minimizing the ecological impact of visitor activities. Ensuring responsible tourism practices, such as designated trails, visitor education, and waste management systems, can help reduce human disturbances and preserve the forest's natural balance.

Promoting Mental Health Education: Educating the public about mental health issues, suicide prevention, and the importance of seeking help is crucial in destigmatizing these topics. Promoting empathy, understanding, and open dialogue can help address the challenges associated with the forest's dark history while fostering a supportive environment.

Collaboration with Mental Health Organizations: Collaborative partnerships between conservation organizations and mental health organizations can provide holistic support for visitors and locals alike. By integrating mental health resources and support into visitor information centers, the stigma surrounding mental health can be addressed while preserving the forest's ecological integrity.

Monitoring and Research: Continuous monitoring and research programs are essential for understanding the forest's ecological dynamics and the impact of human activities. By gathering data on biodiversity, habitat health, and visitor impact, conservation efforts can be adjusted and refined to ensure long-term sustainability.

Invasive Species Management: Invasive species pose a significant threat to the forest's ecological balance. Implementing effective invasive species management programs, such as regular monitoring and removal efforts, helps protect native plant species and maintain the integrity of the forest ecosystem.

Involving Local Communities: Engaging and empowering local communities in conservation efforts is vital. By involving residents in decision-making processes, fostering a sense of ownership, and providing sustainable livelihood opportunities, the local community becomes active stakeholders in preserving the forest's ecological balance.

Education and Awareness: Educating local communities about the importance of ecological conservation, mental health, and sustainable practices helps foster a shared commitment to preserving Aokigahara Forest. Promoting community-based initiatives, such as tree planting campaigns and clean-up activities, strengthens the bond between the community and the forest.

Responsible Media Coverage: Media organizations have a responsibility to report on Aokigahara Forest's dark history with sensitivity and without sensationalism. Promoting responsible media coverage, including ethical guidelines and the inclusion of mental health resources, can help reduce the negative impact of media representation.

Maintaining the ecological balance of Aokigahara Forest while addressing its dark history requires a delicate and thoughtful approach. By prioritizing sensitivity and respect, promoting mental health education, implementing sustainable management practices, engaging local communities, and encouraging responsible media representation, the forest's biodiversity can be preserved while raising awareness about mental health. Balancing the conservation of the forest's natural beauty with addressing its tragic reputation ensures a comprehensive approach that respects both the ecological integrity and the human aspect of Aokigahara Forest.

AOKIGAHARA FOREST: THE HEARTBREAKING SECRETS OF JAPAN'S SUICIDE FOREST

Chapter 10: Navigating the Forest

Exploring Aokigahara Forest can be a unique and enriching experience. However, it is crucial to approach your visit with respect for the environment, the local community, and the forest's history. Here are some practical tips and guidelines to ensure a responsible and meaningful visit:

1. Educate Yourself: Learn about the history, cultural significance, and environmental importance of Aokigahara Forest before your visit. Understanding the context will help you appreciate the forest and its surroundings more deeply.

2. Follow Designated Trails: Stick to designated paths and trails to minimize your impact on the forest. Straying from marked trails can damage fragile vegetation and disrupt wildlife habitats.

3. Leave No Trace: Carry out all your trash and waste. Preserve the forest's natural beauty by keeping it clean and free from litter. Pack reusable water bottles and snacks to minimize waste generation.

4. Respect Wildlife: Observe wildlife from a distance and avoid disturbing or feeding them. Respect their natural behaviors and habitats.

5. Practice Quiet Reflection: Aokigahara Forest is known for its tranquility. Engage in quiet reflection and appreciate the serene environment. Avoid loud conversations, music, or any activities that may disrupt the peaceful ambiance.

6. Do Not Disturb the Environment: Avoid picking or damaging plants, flowers, or any natural elements. Respect the forest's ecosystem and let it thrive undisturbed.

7. Photography and Recording: If taking photographs or recording videos, do so respectfully and without intruding on others' privacy. Be mindful of the forest's solemn reputation and considerate of the experiences of other visitors.

8. Maintain Silence and Reverence: Aokigahara Forest holds a tragic history, and many visit to pay respects to those who have passed away. Maintain a quiet and respectful demeanor, refraining from loud conversations or inappropriate behavior.

9. Be Mindful of Sensitive Areas: Some parts of the forest may hold significance for memorial sites or be more prone to sensitive encounters. Exercise extra caution and respect in these areas.

10. Seek Permission for Filming or Photography: If you plan to engage in professional filming or photography, obtain the necessary permits and permissions in advance. Respect any guidelines or restrictions put in place to protect the forest and its visitors.

11. Be Prepared and Stay Safe: Aokigahara Forest is dense, and navigating through it can be challenging. Ensure you are adequately prepared with appropriate footwear, clothing, and supplies. It is also advisable to inform someone about your visit and expected return time.

12. Consider the Impact of Your Visit: Reflect on the impact your visit may have on the forest and its surroundings. Strive to leave a positive impression and contribute to the conservation efforts aimed at preserving Aokigahara Forest for future generations.

Remember, responsible and respectful behavior is crucial when visiting Aokigahara Forest. By following these guidelines, you can ensure a meaningful and sustainable experience while preserving the forest's ecological balance and cultural significance.

Aokigahara Forest is a unique natural environment, and ensuring safety and responsible tourism practices are essential for both visitors and the preservation of the forest. Here are some insights on safety measures and responsible tourism practices to consider when exploring Aokigahara Forest:

1. Prioritize Personal Safety:

- Plan your visit during daylight hours to ensure better visibility and safety.

- Inform someone about your plans, including your expected duration of stay and intended routes.

- Stay on designated trails and avoid venturing off into dense or dangerous areas.

- Be aware of potential hazards such as unstable terrain, hidden tree roots, and falling branches.

2. Respect the Signage and Regulations:

- Pay attention to warning signs and follow any regulations set by local authorities or conservation organizations.

- Some areas of the forest may be restricted or off-limits. Respect these boundaries to ensure your safety and protect sensitive habitats.

3. Be Prepared and Equipped:

- Wear appropriate clothing and footwear for the forest environment. Comfortable shoes with good traction are recommended.

- Carry essential supplies such as water, snacks, a map or compass, a flashlight, a first aid kit, and a fully charged mobile phone.

- Familiarize yourself with the forest's layout and trail maps to navigate safely.

4. Practice Leave No Trace:

- Follow the principle of "Leave No Trace" by carrying out all trash and waste. Pack a trash bag and dispose of it properly after your visit.

• Avoid disturbing the natural environment by refraining from removing or damaging plants, rocks, or any other natural elements.

5. Maintain Respectful Behavior:

• Be mindful of the forest's reputation and the somber history associated with Aokigahara. Maintain a respectful and solemn demeanor during your visit.

• Keep noise levels low to preserve the tranquility of the forest. Avoid loud conversations, music, or any disruptive activities.

6. Engage in Responsible Photography:

• Respect the privacy of other visitors and be considerate when taking photographs. Ask for permission before photographing individuals or sensitive areas.

• Avoid sharing or posting images that may perpetuate negative stereotypes or sensationalize the forest's reputation.

7. Support Local Conservation Efforts:

• Learn about and support local conservation organizations that work to preserve Aokigahara Forest's ecological integrity and promote responsible tourism practices.

● Consider making a donation to these organizations or participating in volunteer programs that contribute to the forest's conservation.

8. Seek Knowledge and Cultural Understanding:

● Educate yourself about the forest's cultural and historical significance. Understand the local traditions, beliefs, and folklore associated with the forest.

● Engage with local communities respectfully, showing cultural sensitivity and respecting their customs and practices.

9. Contribute to Mental Health Awareness:

● Raise awareness about mental health issues and the importance of seeking help. Share resources and information about mental health support services.

● Advocate for responsible reporting on the forest's history, promoting empathy, understanding, and reducing stigma associated with mental health.

By following these safety measures and responsible tourism practices, you can ensure a safe and meaningful visit to Aokigahara Forest while contributing to the conservation efforts and fostering a positive impact on the environment and local community.

AOKIGAHARA FOREST: THE HEARTBREAKING SECRETS OF JAPAN'S SUICIDE FOREST

Chapter 11: The Psychology of Suicide

Understanding the psychological aspects of suicide is crucial for addressing and preventing this complex phenomenon. This chapter delves into the psychological factors that contribute to suicidal ideation, exploring the intricate web of emotions, mental health conditions, and life circumstances that can play a role.

Depression: Depression is one of the most common mental health conditions associated with suicidal ideation. Feelings of hopelessness, intense sadness, and a distorted perception of reality can contribute to thoughts of self-harm or suicide.

Anxiety Disorders: Individuals with severe anxiety disorders may experience overwhelming fear and a sense of being trapped, leading to feelings of desperation and a desire to escape through suicide.

Bipolar Disorder: The extreme mood swings and intense emotional states experienced in bipolar disorder can increase the risk of suicidal ideation. During depressive episodes, individuals may feel an overwhelming sense of despair and hopelessness.

Substance Abuse: Substance abuse can contribute to suicidal ideation, as it often exacerbates underlying mental health conditions and impairs judgment, increasing feelings of despair and impulsivity.

Hopelessness: A pervasive sense of hopelessness, characterized by a belief that circumstances will never improve, can significantly contribute to suicidal ideation.

Feelings of Isolation: Social isolation and a lack of meaningful connections can lead to feelings of loneliness and despair, increasing the risk of suicidal thoughts.

Shame and Guilt: Intense feelings of shame and guilt, often stemming from past experiences or personal circumstances, can overwhelm individuals and contribute to suicidal ideation.

Emotional Pain and Desperation: Unbearable emotional pain, whether due to traumatic experiences, loss, or ongoing struggles, can drive individuals to consider suicide as a way to escape their suffering.

Relationship Issues: Relationship breakdowns, divorce, or the loss of a loved one can trigger intense emotional distress, leading to thoughts of suicide.

Financial Problems: Overwhelming financial difficulties, such as bankruptcy or job loss, can cause significant stress and contribute to feelings of desperation.

Chronic Physical Illness: Individuals coping with chronic pain or debilitating physical illnesses may experience profound psychological distress, increasing the risk of suicidal ideation.

AOKIGAHARA FOREST: THE HEARTBREAKING SECRETS OF JAPAN'S SUICIDE FOREST

Traumatic Experiences: Past trauma, such as abuse, assault, or witnessing a traumatic event, can have a lasting impact on mental health, contributing to suicidal thoughts.

Perceived Burdensomeness: Some individuals may develop a belief that they are a burden to others, leading to thoughts of self-harm or suicide as a way to relieve others from their perceived burden.

Thwarted Belongingness: The sense of not belonging or feeling disconnected from others can heighten feelings of isolation and contribute to suicidal ideation.

Cognitive Distortions: Negative thought patterns, such as black-and-white thinking, catastrophizing, or persistent self-criticism, can distort perceptions and contribute to hopelessness and suicidal ideation.

Mental Health Treatment: Access to mental health treatment and support services can be instrumental in addressing underlying psychological issues and reducing the risk of suicide.

Social Support: Strong social connections, support networks, and a sense of belonging can act as protective factors, offering emotional support during times of crisis.

Coping Skills: Developing healthy coping mechanisms, problem-solving skills, and resilience can help individuals navigate challenging circumstances and reduce the risk of suicidal ideation.

Suicide Prevention Programs: Education, awareness campaigns, and suicide prevention hotlines play a vital role in providing support, resources, and intervention for individuals in crisis.

Suicidal ideation is a complex issue influenced by a myriad of psychological factors, life circumstances, and emotional experiences. Understanding the psychological aspects of suicide and the contributing factors is essential for effective prevention and support. By addressing mental health conditions, promoting social support, providing access to resources and treatment, and implementing comprehensive suicide prevention strategies, we can work towards reducing the prevalence of suicidal ideation and supporting those in need.

Mental health awareness and support play a critical role in preventing suicide. This chapter explores the significance of promoting mental health awareness, reducing stigma, and providing accessible support systems to individuals at risk of suicide.

Challenging Misconceptions: Increasing mental health awareness involves debunking misconceptions and stereotypes surrounding mental illnesses. Educating the public about the true nature of mental health conditions helps combat stigma and fosters empathy and understanding.

Open Dialogue: Encouraging open and honest conversation about mental health creates a safe space for individuals to share their struggles without fear of judgment or discrimination. I promotes understanding and helps break down the barriers that prevent people from seeking help.

Public Awareness Campaigns: Launching public awareness campaigns raises visibility and educates the general population about mental health issues, warning signs of suicide, and available resources. These campaigns aim to normalize discussions about mental health and empower individuals to seek help when needed.

School-Based Programs: Implementing mental health education programs in schools equips young individuals with knowledge about mental health, coping strategies, and how to seek support. Such initiatives contribute to early intervention and prevention efforts.

Affordable and Accessible Services: Ensuring affordable and accessible mental health services is crucial for individuals in need. Reducing financial barriers, expanding insurance coverage, and increasing the number of mental health professionals help improve access to care and support.

Crisis Hotlines and Helplines: Establishing suicide prevention hotlines and helplines provides individuals with immediate support in times of crisis. These services offer a confidential and empathetic space for individuals to express their thoughts and receive guidance and assistance.

Peer Support Programs: Peer support programs connect individuals with lived experiences of mental health challenges, fostering a sense of belonging and understanding. Peer support offers non-judgmental listening, empathy, and validation, which can be invaluable for individuals in distress.

Supportive Communities: Cultivating supportive communities that prioritize mental health and well-being reduces isolation and creates networks of social support. Encouraging community involvement and fostering a sense of belonging contribute to overall mental health and suicide prevention.

Mental Health Training: Providing comprehensive mental health training for healthcare providers, including primary care physicians, nurses, and psychologists, equips them with the knowledge and skills to identify and respond to individuals at risk of suicide.

Suicide Risk Assessment: Implementing standardized protocols for suicide risk assessment in healthcare settings helps identify individuals in immediate danger and ensures appropriate intervention and support.

Mental health awareness and support are pivotal in preventing suicide and promoting overall well-being. By breaking the stigma, promoting mental health education, enhancing access to mental health services, building support networks, and providing training for healthcare providers, we can create a supportive environment that encourages help-seeking behaviors and early intervention. It is through these efforts that we can work towards reducing the incidence of suicide and ensuring that individuals at risk receive the care, understanding, and support they deserve.

Chapter 12: Scientific Studies and Research

Scientific investigations conducted in Aokigahara Forest have aimed to explore various aspects of the forest's ecosystem, geology, and associated phenomena. While the forest's reputation as a suicide hotspot has garnered significant attention, researchers have also conducted studies to understand its unique characteristics and contribute to broader scientific knowledge. Here are some scientific investigations conducted in Aokigahara Forest:

1. Ecological Studies: Researchers have conducted ecological studies to assess the biodiversity and unique ecosystem within Aokigahara Forest. These studies involve documenting plant and animal species, studying their habitats, and assessing the overall health and conservation status of the forest. By understanding the forest's ecological dynamics, scientists can develop conservation strategies to protect its fragile ecosystem.

2. Geological Surveys: Geological surveys have been conducted to understand the unique geological features and formation of Aokigahara Forest. Scientists have investigated the volcanic origins of the region, mapping out lava flows and studying the impact of volcanic activity on the forest's topography. These surveys provide valuable insights into the forest's geological history and contribute to our understanding of volcanic landscapes.

3. Carbon Cycle Studies: Aokigahara Forest has been the subject of research on carbon cycling and sequestration. Scientists study the forest's ability to absorb and store carbon dioxide, an important factor in mitigating climate change. These studies contribute to our understanding of the role forests play in carbon balance and their potential as carbon sinks.

4. Geomagnetic Anomalies: Some investigations have focused on the presence of geomagnetic anomalies within Aokigahara Forest. Scientists have measured and analyzed magnetic field variations to better understand the underlying geological processes and their potential effects on the forest's ecosystem.

5. Soil Composition and Nutrient Cycling: Researchers have examined the soil composition and nutrient cycling processes in Aokigahara Forest. By studying soil characteristics, such as nutrient content and microbial activity, scientists gain insights into the forest's fertility, plant growth patterns, and overall ecosystem functioning.

6. Lichen Research: Lichens, a symbiotic relationship between fungi and algae, have also been studied in Aokigahara Forest. Lichens are sensitive to environmental changes, and their presence and abundance can provide valuable indicators of air quality and ecosystem health. Research on lichens helps assess the impact of human activities and environmental factors on the forest's ecology.

7. Psychosocial Studies: In addition to ecological research, psychosocial studies have been conducted to understand the mental health aspects associated with Aokigahara Forest. These studies explore the psychological factors contributing to suicidal ideation and aim to develop effective prevention strategies. Researchers investigate the intersection of cultural beliefs, social dynamics, and mental health stigma in the context of the forest.

Scientific investigations in Aokigahara Forest encompass a wide range of disciplines, from ecology and geology to psychology and anthropology. These studies contribute to our understanding of the forest's ecological significance, geological history, and the complex interplay of factors influencing mental health. By conducting rigorous scientific research, we can gain valuable insights into Aokigahara Forest and develop evidence-based strategies for its conservation and the well-being of those who visit or inhabit its surroundings.

Aokigahara Forest has been the subject of several scientific studies across different disciplines, including geology, biology, and psychology. These investigations have provided valuable insights into the unique aspects of the forest. Let's explore some of the key findings from these studies:

Geological Studies:

1. Volcanic Origins: Aokigahara Forest sits atop the Fuji-Hakone-Izu volcanic zone, and geological studies have revealed its origins as a lava flow from past volcanic activity. Researchers have analyzed the composition of volcanic rocks

and lava formations within the forest, shedding light on it geological history.

2. Lava Tube Caves: The forest is also known for its extensiv network of lava tube caves, formed by volcanic eruption Scientific exploration of these caves has uncovered fascinatin geological formations, including stalactites, stalagmites, an lava benches. Studies of these formations contribute to ou understanding of volcanic processes and cave development.

Biology and Ecology Studies:

1. Unique Flora and Fauna: Aokigahara Forest is home to diverse range of plant and animal species that have adapte to the forest's distinct ecological conditions. Studies hav identified unique flora, including mosses, ferns, and variou tree species. The forest also provides habitat for several bir species, small mammals, and insects. Research on the forest biodiversity contributes to conservation efforts and highlight the importance of preserving this unique ecosystem.

2. Decomposition Rates: Due to the forest's dense vegetatio and low human activity, it has become an intriguing locatio for studying decomposition processes. Scientists hav conducted experiments to understand the rates and patterns c decomposition in different environmental conditions withi the forest. These studies contribute to forensic science an ecological research, providing insights into the role c decomposition in nutrient cycling and forest ecosystems.

Psychological Studies:

AOKIGAHARA FOREST: THE HEARTBREAKING SECRETS OF JAPAN'S SUICIDE FOREST

1. Suicidal Ideation and Mental Health: Aokigahara Forest's reputation as a suicide hotspot has prompted psychological research to investigate the factors contributing to suicidal ideation. Studies have examined the relationship between mental health conditions, such as depression and anxiety, and the forest's association with suicidal behavior. These investigations shed light on the complex interplay of psychological factors and the role of environmental context in suicide risk.

2. Cultural Beliefs and Stigma: Psychological studies have explored the cultural beliefs and social stigma surrounding mental health and suicide in Japan, particularly in relation to Aokigahara Forest. Researchers have examined the impact of cultural and societal factors on help-seeking behaviors and the challenges in addressing mental health issues. These studies provide insights into the intersection of culture, mental health, and suicide prevention strategies.

By integrating geology, biology, and psychology, scientists have deepened our understanding of Aokigahara Forest. These studies have highlighted the forest's geological origins, unique flora and fauna, and the complex psychological factors associated with its reputation. Through ongoing research and interdisciplinary collaborations, scientists continue to uncover the intricate and multifaceted aspects of this enigmatic forest, contributing to its conservation and informing strategies for mental health support and suicide prevention.

Chapter 13: Healing and Transformation

While Aokigahara Forest is primarily known for its association with suicide and dark legends, there are alternative perspectives that view the forest as a place of healing and personal growth. These perspectives emphasize the forest's serene environment, natural beauty, and spiritual significance, offering individuals an opportunity for reflection, introspection, and self-discovery. Here are some alternative viewpoints on Aokigahara Forest:

1. Nature's Therapeutic Power: Supporters of this perspective believe that connecting with nature can have a profound healing effect on the mind, body, and spirit. Aokigahara Forest, with its tranquil atmosphere, lush greenery, and calming sounds, provides a serene backdrop for individuals seeking solace and a sense of rejuvenation.

2. Contemplative Space: Some individuals see Aokigahara Forest as a contemplative space, ideal for introspection and self-reflection. The forest's quietude, coupled with its ancient trees and secluded pathways, creates an ambiance that encourages deep thought and personal growth.

3. Connection with Ancient Traditions: Aokigahara Forest holds cultural and spiritual significance in Japanese folklore and traditions. For those who appreciate these beliefs, the forest can be seen as a place to connect with ancestral roots, seek spiritual insights, or engage in rituals that promote personal healing and transformation.

4. Symbolism of Renewal: Advocates of this viewpoint view Aokigahara Forest as a symbol of renewal and resilience. Despite its dark reputation, the forest has continued to thrive and adapt throughout history. Some individuals find inspiration in this resilience, perceiving the forest as a metaphor for their own ability to overcome challenges and grow stronger.

5. Artistic Inspiration: Aokigahara Forest's unique atmosphere and haunting beauty have inspired artists, writers, and photographers. They see the forest as a muse, drawing upon its ethereal qualities to create meaningful works of art that explore themes of introspection, mortality, and the human experience.

6. Symbolic Transformation: The forest's association with death and darkness can be reframed as a symbolic representation of personal transformation. Some individuals view Aokigahara Forest as a place to confront their inner demons, confront past traumas, and emerge stronger, akin to the forest's ability to regenerate and flourish despite its tragic history.

It is important to approach these alternative perspectives with sensitivity and respect, recognizing that individual experiences and interpretations may vary. While these perspectives shed light on the potential for healing and personal growth within Aokigahara Forest, it is essential to acknowledge the forest's

AOKIGAHARA FOREST: THE HEARTBREAKING SECRETS OF JAPAN'S SUICIDE FOREST

complex history and the importance of promoting mental health awareness and suicide prevention in any discussion related to the forest.

Transforming Aokigahara Forest's reputation and promoting mental well-being requires a multi-faceted approach that involves various stakeholders, including government bodies, local communities, mental health organizations, and the general public. Here are some potential strategies for transforming the forest's reputation and promoting mental well-being:

1. Awareness and Education:

> • Develop comprehensive mental health awareness campaigns that focus on reducing stigma and promoting understanding of mental health issues.

> • Provide accurate information about Aokigahara Forest, including its natural beauty, ecological significance, and cultural history, to challenge misconceptions and stereotypes.

> • Offer educational programs in schools and communities to raise awareness about mental health, suicide prevention, and the importance of seeking help.

2. Enhanced Mental Health Support:

● Increase access to mental health services, including counseling, therapy, and support groups, in the local area surrounding Aokigahara Forest.

● Collaborate with mental health organizations to establish crisis hotlines, helplines, or mobile support units that can offer immediate assistance to individuals in distress.

● Train local healthcare providers and volunteers in suicide prevention, risk assessment, and intervention techniques.

3. Environmental Conservation and Restoration:

● Implement conservation efforts to protect the unique ecosystem of Aokigahara Forest, highlighting its ecological importance and encouraging sustainable practices.

● Organize community-led initiatives for reforestation, habitat restoration, and clean-up campaigns, fostering a sense of stewardship and connection to the forest's natural beauty.

4. Alternative Uses and Activities:

● Promote the forest's potential for recreational and therapeutic activities, such as nature walks, guided tours, mindfulness retreats, and outdoor workshops.

● Encourage the establishment of visitor centers or information hubs that provide educational resources, mental health support information, and guidance for responsible forest exploration.

5. Collaboration and Partnerships:

● Foster collaboration between local communities, mental health organizations, conservation groups, and government agencies to develop integrated strategies for promoting mental well-being and sustainable forest management.

● Engage with researchers, psychologists, and sociologists to conduct studies on the positive aspects of Aokigahara Forest, such as its potential for healing, resilience, and personal growth.

6. Responsible Media Coverage:

● Encourage responsible media reporting that emphasizes mental health awareness, positive narratives, and respectful portrayal of Aokigahara Forest.

● Provide guidelines and training for journalists and content creators to ensure accurate, sensitive, and ethical reporting on topics related to the forest and mental health.

It is important to approach these initiatives with cultural sensitivity, respect for the forest's history, and a commitment to collaborative decision-making involving local communities. By addressing the forest's reputation, promoting mental well-being, and fostering a deeper understanding of the forest's unique attributes, we can transform Aokigahara Forest into a place that not only respects its natural beauty but also promotes healing, personal growth, and mental well-being for all who visit.

AOKIGAHARA FOREST: THE HEARTBREAKING SECRETS OF JAPAN'S SUICIDE FOREST

Chapter 14: Forest Folklore and Ghost Stories

Aokigahara Forest, with its enigmatic ambiance and haunting reputation, has spawned eerie tales and ghostly legends over the years. While it's important to approach these stories with skepticism and cultural sensitivity, they add to the mystique surrounding the forest. Here are some of the eerie tales and ghostly legends associated with Aokigahara Forest:

1. **Yurei:** Aokigahara Forest is believed to be inhabited by yurei, vengeful spirits of the deceased. According to legend, these spirits linger in the forest, their anguished souls trapped between the realms of the living and the dead. Some claim to have heard disembodied voices or seen apparitions while wandering through the dense vegetation.

2. **Ghostly Encounters:** Visitors have reported strange encounters within Aokigahara Forest. Witnesses claim to have seen shadowy figures darting between trees, felt cold spots, or experienced an overwhelming feeling of being watched. Some believe these encounters are the result of the forest's dark history and the lingering energy associated with tragic events.

3. **Mysterious Disappearances:** Aokigahara Forest has gained a reputation for mysterious disappearances. It is said that once someone enters the forest, they may never return. Legends suggest that malevolent spirits or supernatural forces within

the forest lure wanderers astray, making it difficult for them to find their way back.

4. The Wailing Forest: Local folklore describes Aokigahara Forest as a place where anguished cries and eerie wails can be heard during the night. These haunting sounds are believed to be the voices of the lost souls trapped within the forest, crying out for release or seeking to lure others to their fate.

5. Cursed Grounds: Some legends suggest that Aokigahara Forest is cursed or holds a dark energy. It is believed that negative energy accumulates within the forest due to the tragic events that have occurred there, leading to an eerie and unsettling atmosphere that is palpable to those who venture into its depths.

6. Aokigahara Forest Guide: According to local tales, there are individuals known as "Aokigahara Forest Guides" who possess supernatural abilities to navigate the forest. These guides are said to be able to communicate with spirits, providing protection and guidance to those who seek their assistance in navigating the labyrinthine trails.

While these eerie tales and ghostly legends contribute to the fascination surrounding Aokigahara Forest, it is important to approach them with a critical mindset and respect for the cultural context. The forest's reputation should not overshadow the need for mental health awareness, suicide prevention, and responsible exploration of this unique natural environment.

AOKIGAHARA FOREST: THE HEARTBREAKING SECRETS OF JAPAN'S SUICIDE FOREST

The cultural fascination with supernatural phenomena in the context of Aokigahara Forest can be attributed to a combination of factors, including folklore, historical events, psychological intrigue, and the human fascination with the mysterious and unexplained. Here is an analysis of the cultural fascination with supernatural phenomena in relation to Aokigahara Forest:

1. Folklore and Legends: Japanese folklore is rich with tales of spirits, ghosts, and supernatural beings. Aokigahara Forest's association with yurei (vengeful spirits) and ghostly encounters taps into this longstanding cultural belief in the existence of otherworldly entities. These legends provide a framework for interpreting and understanding the unexplained phenomena reported in the forest.

2. Historical Tragedies: Aokigahara Forest's reputation as a suicide hotspot and its historical association with the practice of ubasute (a form of abandoning the elderly) contribute to the sense of tragedy and darkness that surrounds the forest. Such historical events create a fertile ground for the development of supernatural narratives and stories that attempt to explain the eerie atmosphere and strange occurrences within the forest.

3. Psychological Intrigue: The eerie ambiance of Aokigahara Forest, with its dense vegetation, quietude, and stark contrasts, evokes a sense of psychological intrigue. The forest's association with death and despair draws curiosity and sparks the human imagination, prompting contemplation about the mysteries of life, mortality, and the afterlife. This fascination with the human psyche and the exploration of existential questions fuels the cultural fascination with supernatural phenomena.

4. Media Representation: Aokigahara Forest's reputation as the "Suicide Forest" has garnered significant attention in books, films, documentaries, and online content. Media representation amplifies the forest's mystique, perpetuating its association with supernatural elements and contributing to public curiosity and fascination. This media exposure further reinforces the cultural fascination with the forest's supernatural phenomena.

5. Thrill-Seeking and Adventure: For some individuals, the allure of supernatural phenomena lies in the thrill and excitement of exploring the unknown. Aokigahara Forest's reputation as an eerie and haunted location attracts thrill-seekers, adventure enthusiasts, and paranormal investigators who are drawn to the possibility of encountering supernatural entities or witnessing unexplained phenomena.

It is important to note that while cultural fascination with supernatural phenomena in the context of Aokigahara Forest exists, it should be approached with sensitivity and respect. The forest's association with suicide and mental health issues calls for a balanced perspective that prioritizes mental health awareness, compassion, and responsible exploration, rather than solely focusing on the sensationalized aspects of the supernatural.

AOKIGAHARA FOREST: THE HEARTBREAKING SECRETS OF JAPAN'S SUICIDE FOREST

Chapter 15: Filmmaking and Media Influence

A okigahara Forest has been the subject of various movies, documentaries, and other media, each portraying the forest in different ways. These portrayals have both sparked public interest and generated controversy due to the sensitive nature of the forest's reputation. Here is an exploration of the portrayal of Aokigahara Forest in different forms of media:

1. Movies:

- "The Sea of Trees" (2015): This drama film directed by Gus Van Sant tells the story of a man who travels to Aokigahara Forest with the intention of ending his life but encounters another lost soul. The film explores themes of redemption and the search for meaning amid despair, though it drew criticism for its handling of the sensitive topic and for utilizing the forest as a backdrop for a fictional narrative.

- "The Forest" (2016): A horror film set in Aokigahara Forest, "The Forest" follows a woman searching for her missing twin sister who is believed to have entered the forest. The movie portrays the forest as a malevolent entity that plays on people's fears and psychological vulnerabilities. While the film attracted attention for its horror elements, it also faced backlash for capitalizing on the forest's tragic reputation.

2. Documentaries:

- "Aokigahara: Suicide Forest" (2011): This documentary by VICE News explores the forest's association with suicide and the challenges faced by local authorities and volunteers who work to prevent self-harm. It provides an in-depth look into the cultural and psychological factors contributing to the forest's reputation.

- "The Departed Souls: Aokigahara" (2019): Directed by Youtuber Nux Taku, this documentary-style video offers a mix of exploration, folklore, and personal reflections on Aokigahara Forest. It attempts to showcase the forest's natural beauty while acknowledging its tragic history.

3. Online Media and Articles:

- Internet Content: Aokigahara Forest has gained significant attention on social media platforms and online forums, with individuals sharing their experiences, photos, and stories related to the forest. Some content creators use Aokigahara Forest as a backdrop for horror-themed videos, while others strive to raise awareness about mental health and suicide prevention.

AOKIGAHARA FOREST: THE HEARTBREAKING SECRETS OF JAPAN'S SUICIDE FOREST

● News Articles: Various news outlets have reported on Aokigahara Forest, often highlighting its association with suicide and exploring the efforts to raise awareness and prevent self-harm. These articles play a crucial role in informing the public about the complexities of the forest's reputation and the importance of addressing mental health issues.

It is important to approach portrayals of Aokigahara Forest in movies, documentaries, and other media with critical thinking and cultural sensitivity. While media coverage can help shed light on the forest's complexities, it should prioritize responsible reporting, accurate information, and empathy towards individuals affected by mental health challenges. The forest's reputation should not overshadow the need for mental health awareness, suicide prevention, and respectful engagement with this unique natural environment.

The media plays a significant role in shaping public perception, including how places like Aokigahara Forest are portrayed and understood. However, there are important ethical implications and responsibilities that the media must consider when covering sensitive topics and locations:

1. Sensationalism and Exploitation: Media outlets should avoid sensationalizing tragedies or exploiting sensitive subjects for the sake of generating attention or profit. Sensationalized coverage can perpetuate harmful stereotypes, reinforce stigmas, and potentially glamorize or romanticize harmful behaviors. Responsible reporting should prioritize empathy, accuracy, and a nuanced understanding of the complex issues at hand.

2. Privacy and Sensitivity: Media coverage should respect the privacy and dignity of individuals affected by tragic events or mental health struggles. Care should be taken to avoid identifying specific individuals or sharing graphic details that can further traumatize families and communities. Sensitivity to the emotions and vulnerabilities of those involved is crucial in maintaining ethical journalistic standards.

3. Balancing Public Interest and Responsibility: While public interest in certain topics is natural, media outlets should exercise responsibility in presenting information that is accurate, well-researched, and fair. This includes providing context, offering diverse perspectives, and avoiding the perpetuation of stereotypes or biased narratives that may lead to misrepresentation or misunderstanding.

4. Promoting Mental Health Awareness and Resources: The media has the power to educate and inform the public about mental health issues, including suicide prevention, available resources, and the importance of seeking help. Coverage should prioritize accurate information, provide helpline numbers, and highlight stories of recovery and resilience. This can help reduce stigma, provide support, and offer a more balanced understanding of complex topics.

5. Collaborative Approaches and Dialogue: Engaging with mental health experts, researchers, and community organizations can help ensure that media coverage is well-informed and inclusive. Collaborative approaches foster a deeper understanding of the issues at hand, allow for diverse perspectives to be shared, and create opportunities for constructive dialogue that promotes accuracy and ethical reporting.

6. Long-term Impact: Media coverage can have lasting effects on public perception and the individuals involved. Journalists and media professionals should consider the potential consequences of their coverage and strive to provide balanced, responsible reporting that contributes positively to public discourse, understanding, and societal well-being.

By adhering to ethical principles and responsibilities, the media can play a crucial role in shaping public perception in a responsible and respectful manner. Thoughtful and sensitive coverage contributes to informed discussions, increased awareness, and more compassionate approaches to complex topics like mental health and sensitive locations like Aokigahara Forest.

OLIVER LANCASTER

Chapter 16: Environmental Impact

Tourism and human activity in Aokigahara Forest have had a significant impact on its delicate ecosystem. While the forest is known for its natural beauty and cultural significance, the increase in visitors and related activities has presented various challenges. Here are some key impacts of tourism and human activity on the forest's ecosystem:

1. Vegetation Damage: Unregulated tourism and human activity can lead to trampling, habitat destruction, and damage to vegetation. Paths created by visitors deviating from designated trails can disrupt the natural growth patterns of plants and disrupt the forest's ecological balance.

2. Soil Erosion: Excessive foot traffic and off-trail exploration can accelerate soil erosion, particularly in sensitive areas. Loss of vegetation cover and compaction of soil disrupt the natural processes that promote soil fertility and stability. Erosion can also result in the sedimentation of nearby water bodies, affecting aquatic ecosystems.

3. Disturbance of Wildlife: Frequent human presence and activities can disturb wildlife, leading to changes in their behavior, breeding patterns, and foraging activities. Animals may be displaced from their natural habitats or become habituated to human presence, altering their natural ecological interactions.

4. Trash and Pollution: Increased tourism often brings with it an influx of visitors who may not prioritize responsible waste management. Littering and improper disposal of trash can degrade the forest environment and pose risks to wildlife. Pollution from plastics, chemicals, and other waste materials can contaminate soil, water bodies, and the overall ecosystem.

5. Invasive Species Introduction: Human activity, including the introduction of non-native plant species, can disrupt the natural balance of the forest. Invasive species can outcompete native vegetation, reducing biodiversity and altering the habitat structure. This can have cascading effects on other organisms dependent on native flora for food and shelter.

6. Fire Risks: Human activity, such as the use of open flame for camping or negligence with cigarette disposal, increase the risk of forest fires. Fires can lead to extensive damage, destroying vegetation, disrupting wildlife habitats, and altering the forest's natural regeneration processes.

Mitigating the Impact:

- Implementing visitor management strategies, such as designated trails, visitor education programs, and limiting visitor numbers, can help minimize damage to the forest ecosystem.

- Enforcing regulations against littering and irresponsible behavior through increased monitoring and awareness campaigns.

● Promoting responsible tourism practices, including packing out all waste, adhering to designated trails, and respecting wildlife and vegetation.

● Engaging local communities and stakeholders in conservation efforts, fostering a sense of stewardship and involvement in protecting the forest's ecosystem.

● Conducting ongoing research and monitoring to assess the ecological impacts of human activity and inform sustainable management practices.

By recognizing the potential impact of tourism and human activity on Aokigahara Forest's ecosystem and implementing responsible practices, we can strive to preserve its natural beauty, protect its biodiversity, and maintain its cultural significance for future generations.

Efforts to mitigate environmental damage and restore the natural balance in Aokigahara Forest have been undertaken by various organizations, local communities, and government bodies. These initiatives aim to address the impacts of tourism and human activity while promoting the long-term conservation of the forest's ecosystem. Here are some key efforts in this regard:

1. Reforestation and Habitat Restoration: Organizations and community groups have been actively involved in reforestation projects to restore areas of the forest that have been damaged or depleted. These initiatives involve planting native tree species and ensuring proper habitat restoration to encourage the recovery of the forest ecosystem.

2. Visitor Education and Awareness: Efforts to raise awareness among visitors about responsible tourism practices and the importance of preserving the forest's ecosystem have been implemented. Informational signage, guided tours, and educational programs emphasize the need to stay on designated trails, properly dispose of waste, and respect the flora and fauna.

3. Sustainable Tourism Practices: Collaborative efforts between local communities, tour operators, and government agencies have focused on promoting sustainable tourism practices. These initiatives include setting visitor limits, regulating access to sensitive areas, and encouraging eco-friendly activities that minimize the impact on the forest's ecosystem.

4. Waste Management and Cleanup Campaigns: Regular cleanup campaigns involving volunteers and local communities have been organized to remove litter and debris from the forest. These initiatives aim to minimize pollution, protect wildlife, and create a cleaner environment for both visitors and the ecosystem.

5. Research and Monitoring: Ongoing research and monitoring efforts provide valuable data on the forest's ecological health, helping to identify areas of concern and guide conservation strategies. This includes studying vegetation recovery, wildlife populations, and the impact of human activity on the forest ecosystem.

6. Collaborative Conservation Partnerships: Collaboration between government agencies, research institutions, local communities, and non-profit organizations plays a crucial role in implementing conservation measures. These partnerships facilitate the sharing of knowledge, resources, and expertise, leading to more effective conservation strategies and sustainable management practices.

7. Enforcement of Regulations: The enforcement of regulations and guidelines pertaining to forest conservation and responsible visitation is important in preserving the natural balance of the forest. Park rangers and forest officials work to ensure compliance with rules, prevent illegal activities, and protect sensitive areas within the forest.

By combining these efforts, there is a growing commitment to mitigating environmental damage and restoring the natural balance in Aokigahara Forest. These initiatives aim to create a sustainable framework that allows visitors to appreciate the forest's beauty while preserving its fragile ecosystem for future generations. Continued collaboration, research, and community engagement are vital in ensuring the long-term conservation and restoration of Aokigahara Forest.

Chapter 17: Indigenous Wisdom and Practices

Aokigahara Forest, located in Japan, is not traditionally associated with specific indigenous beliefs and practices. However, it is important to recognize and respect the Ainu people, the indigenous inhabitants of Hokkaido, and their spiritual connections to the land and forests in the region. While the Ainu's direct connection to Aokigahara Forest specifically may not be well-documented, their broader cultural beliefs regarding forests and nature provide valuable insights into indigenous perspectives. Here are some key aspects to consider:

1. **Animistic Beliefs:** The Ainu traditionally follow an animistic belief system, perceiving spirits or deities known as "kamuy" in natural elements, including forests, rivers, and mountains. They believe that these spiritual beings possess a life force and play a significant role in their lives. The forest, as a part of nature, is likely to hold significance in their spiritual worldview.

2. **Spiritual Connection to Nature:** Indigenous cultures often emphasize a profound connection with the natural world, including forests. The Ainu people are known for their deep reverence for nature and their reliance on the forest for sustenance, materials, and cultural practices. They see

themselves as part of a larger ecosystem, living in harmony with the land and its resources.

3. Rituals and Ceremonies: Indigenous cultures typically have specific rituals and ceremonies to honor and express gratitude to the land and its spiritual beings. Although specific rituals related to Aokigahara Forest are not known, the Ainu likely have ceremonies and practices associated with forests in general. These ceremonies may involve offerings, prayers, dances, and songs to establish and maintain a harmonious relationship with the forest and its spiritual entities.

4. Cultural Heritage: The Ainu have a rich cultural heritage that encompasses traditional knowledge, crafts, and practices related to their connection with the natural world. Their expertise in utilizing forest resources for food, medicine, clothing, and housing reflects their profound understanding of the forest ecosystem and their sustainable practices.

While specific information about the Ainu's connection to Aokigahara Forest is limited, their overall cultural beliefs and practices provide insights into indigenous perspectives on forests and their spiritual significance. It is crucial to approach and interpret indigenous beliefs and practices with respect, seeking to learn from and amplify indigenous voices and perspectives when discussing Aokigahara Forest or any other indigenous lands.

Aokigahara Forest holds wisdom and spiritual significance for local communities in Japan. While not exclusive to indigenous communities, the forest's cultural and historical context has shaped its significance for those who reside in the region. Here are some aspects of the wisdom and spiritual significance attached to Aokigahara Forest by local communities:

1. Cultural Heritage and Connection: Aokigahara Forest is deeply intertwined with the cultural heritage of Japan. Its ancient trees, tranquil atmosphere, and rich biodiversity evoke a sense of reverence and respect among local communities. The forest is often viewed as a sacred place, reflecting a long-standing connection between the land and its people.

2. Symbolism of Renewal and Resilience: Despite its association with tragedy, Aokigahara Forest embodies the resilience of nature. The ability of the forest to regenerate, grow, and thrive despite its dark history is seen as a symbol of renewal and strength. This resilience is often attributed to the wisdom inherent in nature, teaching lessons of adaptability and the cyclical nature of life.

3. Nature's Healing Power: Aokigahara Forest is recognized as a place of solace and healing. The serene environment, surrounded by lush greenery, is believed to offer comfort and tranquility to those seeking solace or a connection with the natural world. Local communities value the forest as a sanctuary where individuals can find respite from the stresses of daily life.

4. Spiritual Reflection and Introspection: The forest's dense vegetation, quietude, and mystical atmosphere inspire introspection and self-reflection. It is seen as a space where individuals can engage in contemplation, reconnect with their inner selves, and seek spiritual insights. The forest's natural beauty is believed to provide a backdrop for deep thought, personal growth, and a sense of unity with the larger universe.

5. Cultural Practices and Rituals: Local communities may engage in cultural practices and rituals associated with Aokigahara Forest. These may include offerings to spirits or deities, prayers for protection and guidance, or ceremonies to honor the forest and its spiritual significance. These practices foster a sense of connection, tradition, and continuity with the land and its spiritual heritage.

6. Environmental Stewardship: The local communities surrounding Aokigahara Forest often have a deep appreciation for its ecological value and actively engage in environmental stewardship. They understand the importance of preserving the forest's biodiversity, protecting its delicate ecosystem, and promoting sustainable practices to ensure its long-term well-being.

It is important to note that the wisdom and spiritual significance attached to Aokigahara Forest may vary among different individuals and communities. While some may emphasize cultural traditions and spiritual connections, others may appreciate the forest's beauty and ecological importance. Understanding and respecting these diverse perspectives contribute to a holistic appreciation of the forest's wisdom and spiritual significance for local communities.

AOKIGAHARA FOREST: THE HEARTBREAKING SECRETS OF JAPAN'S SUICIDE FOREST

Chapter 18: Reflecting on Aokigahara

Throughout the book, we have delved into the mystique, history, and cultural significance of Aokigahara Forest. We have explored the forest's reputation as the "Suicide Forest," its connection to Japanese folklore, and the unique geological features that shape its landscape. We have also examined the impact of human activity on the forest's ecosystem, the stories and legends associated with it, and the efforts to preserve its natural balance while addressing its dark history.

As I reflect on the themes and stories explored, a profound sense of complexity emerges. Aokigahara Forest is a place of contrasts, where beauty intertwines with tragedy, and mystery meets human experience. The forest's reputation as a suicide hotspot brings to light the fragile nature of mental health and the universal human struggle to find meaning and solace in the face of despair.

The stories of those who have ventured into the forest have left a lasting impact. From personal accounts of survival and encounters with the supernatural, to emotional journeys of introspection and growth, these narratives remind us of the immense power of nature and the resilience of the human spirit. They also serve as a poignant reminder of the importance of mental health awareness and support systems that can offer hope and help in times of darkness.

Exploring the indigenous beliefs and spiritual significance attached to the forest, we are reminded of the deep wisdom and interconnectedness of nature and humanity. The forest holds lessons of renewal, resilience, and the potential for personal transformation. It serves as a sanctuary for reflection, a place where individuals can find solace, seek spiritual insights, and reconnect with themselves and the natural world.

While Aokigahara Forest has been a subject of fascination and intrigue, it is essential to approach its stories and themes with sensitivity, respect, and a commitment to understanding the broader context of mental health and the cultural heritage of the region. Through responsible engagement and open dialogue, we can continue to shed light on the complex layers of this enigmatic forest while promoting empathy, mental well-being, and environmental stewardship.

May the stories and reflections within this book inspire greater compassion, awareness, and action—encouraging us to confront the challenges surrounding mental health, celebrate the wisdom of nature, and embrace the potential for healing and growth even in the darkest of places. Let us carry these lessons forward as we navigate our own journeys and contribute to a more understanding and compassionate world.

As you journey through the exploration of Aokigahara Forest, I encourage you to reflect upon your own perceptions and reactions to this enigmatic place. Recognize that the forest reputation as the "Suicide Forest" has shaped its public image, but there is much more to discover beyond the surface.

AOKIGAHARA FOREST: THE HEARTBREAKING SECRETS OF JAPAN'S SUICIDE FOREST

Consider the power of storytelling and the influence of media in shaping our understanding. How have your preconceived notions been challenged or reinforced by the stories shared within these pages? Are there biases or assumptions that you bring to your exploration of Aokigahara Forest? Take a moment to critically examine these perspectives and be open to new insights.

Contemplate the impact of mental health and the importance of empathy and support. Aokigahara Forest serves as a stark reminder of the struggles faced by individuals in their darkest moments. How does this realization deepen your understanding of mental health issues? How can you contribute to creating a more compassionate and supportive society for those in need?

Explore your connection to nature and the healing power it holds. As you read about the forest's spiritual significance and its capacity to inspire personal growth, consider your own relationship with the natural world. How does nature impact your well-being? How can you cultivate a deeper appreciation for the natural environments around you?

Challenge the stereotypes and stigmas surrounding Aokigahara Forest. While acknowledging the forest's tragic history, strive to see beyond its reputation. Recognize the complexities of this place and the individuals who are drawn to it. How can we move beyond simplistic narratives and foster a more nuanced understanding of Aokigahara Forest and the broader issues it represents?

Ultimately, I encourage you to approach your exploration of Aokigahara Forest with an open mind, empathy, and respect. Engage in conversations, seek diverse perspectives, and question the narratives that have shaped our perceptions. By doing so, you contribute to a deeper understanding of the forest, mental health, and the importance of compassion in our interactions with one another.

May your journey through the stories and themes of Aokigahara Forest ignite a sense of curiosity, reflection, and empathy within you. Let it inspire you to think critically, challenge assumptions, and foster a greater appreciation for the complexities of the human experience and the natural world that surrounds us.

AOKIGAHARA FOREST: THE HEARTBREAKING SECRETS OF JAPAN'S SUICIDE FOREST

Chapter 19: Looking Ahead

The future of Aokigahara Forest holds both challenges and opportunities as its evolving role in Japanese society continues to unfold. Here are some key considerations:

1. Conservation and Sustainability: As the forest's reputation draws increased attention, it is crucial to prioritize its conservation and sustainability. Efforts to mitigate environmental damage, restore the natural balance, and implement responsible tourism practices should be strengthened. This includes ongoing research, collaboration with local communities, and the adoption of sustainable management strategies to ensure the long-term health of the forest ecosystem.

2. Mental Health Awareness and Suicide Prevention: Aokigahara Forest has become a symbol of the profound challenges faced by individuals dealing with mental health issues. Its evolving role in Japanese society should be coupled with a heightened focus on mental health awareness, suicide prevention, and support services. This includes fostering open conversations, reducing stigma, and ensuring accessible resources for those in need.

3. Cultural Understanding and Sensitivity: As Aokigahara Forest's reputation continues to evolve, it is crucial to promote cultural understanding and sensitivity. This involves recognizing the forest's cultural significance within the broader context of Japanese folklore, indigenous beliefs, and spiritual practices. Embracing diverse perspectives and engaging in respectful dialogue can lead to a more nuanced understanding of the forest's role in Japanese society.

4. Research and Education: Continued research and education about Aokigahara Forest can contribute to a deeper understanding of its geological, ecological, and cultural aspects. Encouraging interdisciplinary studies, supporting academic research, and providing educational resources can foster a more informed and balanced perspective on the forest's significance and challenges.

5. Community Engagement and Collaboration: Collaboration between government agencies, local communities, non-profit organizations, and other stakeholders is vital for shaping the future of Aokigahara Forest. Engaging with local communities, respecting their knowledge and experiences, and involving them in decision-making processes ensures that their voices are heard and their interests are considered in sustainable forest management.

6. Evolving Cultural Narratives: Aokigahara Forest's evolving role in Japanese society may involve a shift in cultural narratives. Beyond its association with tragedy, there is potential for highlighting the forest's natural beauty, biodiversity, and potential for personal growth and healing. This shift can contribute to a more balanced and positive perception of the forest, emphasizing its broader value beyond its dark history.

By considering these aspects, we can work towards a future for Aokigahara Forest that encompasses conservation, mental health support, cultural understanding, and sustainable practices. The forest's evolving role in Japanese society presents an opportunity to promote healing, resilience, and a greater appreciation for the complexities of nature and the human experience.

Addressing mental health and suicide prevention in the region surrounding Aokigahara Forest requires a multifaceted approach involving various stakeholders. Here are potential strategies that can contribute to these efforts:

1. Awareness and Education: Promote widespread awareness and education about mental health, including the signs of distress, available resources, and destigmatization. Implement campaigns that encourage open conversations, challenge societal norms around mental health, and promote help-seeking behavior.

2. Mental Health Services: Improve access to mental health services, including counseling, therapy, and crisis hotlines. Increase funding for mental health programs and ensure that services are available to individuals in need, particularly in rural areas where resources may be limited.

3. Community Support and Outreach: Develop community-based programs that provide support networks and safe spaces for individuals struggling with mental health issues. Foster collaboration between local organizations, healthcare providers, and community leaders to promote community engagement and a sense of belonging.

4. Training and Capacity Building: Provide training and capacity-building initiatives for healthcare professionals, educators, community leaders, and volunteers on mental health awareness, suicide prevention, and intervention strategies. Empower these individuals to recognize warning signs, offer support, and refer individuals to appropriate services.

5. Early Intervention and Screening: Implement early intervention programs in schools, workplaces, and other community settings to identify individuals at risk and provide timely support. Encourage mental health screenings and assessments to ensure early detection and intervention for those in need.

6. Collaboration with Indigenous Communities: Collaborate with indigenous communities, such as the Ainu, to incorporate their cultural wisdom and practices into mental health and suicide prevention strategies. Engage in respectful dialogue, learn from their experiences, and incorporate indigenous perspectives on well-being and connection with nature.

7. Research and Data Collection: Promote research on mental health, suicide prevention, and the specific factors contributing to distress in the region. Collect data to inform evidence-based interventions, identify high-risk populations, and evaluate the effectiveness of prevention efforts.

8. Media Guidelines and Responsible Reporting: Develop media guidelines for reporting on mental health and suicide-related topics, promoting responsible and ethical coverage. Encourage journalists and media outlets to prioritize accurate information, avoid sensationalism, and provide resources for individuals seeking help.

9. Collaboration between Government and NGOs: Foster collaboration between government agencies, non-governmental organizations (NGOs), and community-based organizations to develop comprehensive mental health policies, coordinate resources, and implement prevention programs effectively.

10. International Cooperation: Promote international cooperation and knowledge-sharing on mental health and suicide prevention strategies. Collaborate with global organizations and draw upon international best practices to develop comprehensive approaches tailored to the local context.

By implementing these strategies, it is possible to create a supportive environment that prioritizes mental health, reduces stigma, and provides the necessary resources and interventions to prevent suicide. It requires a collective effort from individuals, communities, government entities, and relevant organizations to address mental health challenges effectively and support the well-being of those in the region.

Chapter 20: Lessons from Aokigahara Forest

1. **Complexity and Contrasts:** Aokigahara Forest is a place of complexity, where beauty and tragedy coexist. Its reputation as the "Suicide Forest" highlights the profound challenges faced by individuals dealing with mental health issues, while its natural beauty and cultural significance evoke a sense of reverence and connection.

2. **Mental Health Awareness:** The forest's association with suicide calls for increased mental health awareness and support. It is essential to foster open conversations, reduce stigma, and provide accessible resources to promote well-being and prevent suicide.

3. **Cultural Significance:** Aokigahara Forest holds cultural significance within the broader context of Japanese folklore and indigenous beliefs. It is a place of spiritual reflection, personal growth, and connection to nature. Understanding and respecting these cultural aspects contribute to a deeper appreciation of the forest's role in Japanese society.

4. **Environmental Conservation:** The forest's delicate ecosystem requires conservation efforts and sustainable practices. Mitigating environmental damage, promoting responsible tourism, and restoring the natural balance are crucial for preserving the forest's biodiversity and long-term health.

5. Ethical Responsibility: Media and individuals have an ethical responsibility to approach Aokigahara Forest with sensitivity, respect, and a commitment to understanding the broader context of mental health and cultural heritage. Responsible reporting, compassion, and cultural sensitivity are essential in shaping public perception.

6. Personal Reflection: Engaging with Aokigahara Forest invites personal reflection on our own perceptions, biases, and connections to nature. It encourages us to question assumptions, deepen our understanding of mental health issues, and cultivate empathy towards others' struggles.

7. Collaborative Approaches: Addressing the challenges associated with Aokigahara Forest requires collaboration between stakeholders, including government agencies, local communities, non-profit organizations, and researchers. Engaging in dialogue, sharing knowledge, and working together fosters comprehensive approaches and sustainable solutions.

By considering these key takeaways, we can foster greater understanding, compassion, and environmental stewardship. Aokigahara Forest serves as a reminder of the interconnectedness between mental health, cultural beliefs, and the natural world. Through responsible engagement and collective efforts, we can promote mental well-being, cultural appreciation, and the conservation of this enigmatic forest.

As you conclude your journey through the exploration of Aokigahara Forest and its complex themes, I encourage you to continue the conversation and take action to promote mental well-being in your own life and beyond. Here are some ways to keep the dialogue alive and make a positive impact:

1. Foster Open Conversations: Engage in conversations about mental health with friends, family, and colleagues. Create a safe and non-judgmental space where people feel comfortable sharing their experiences, challenges, and emotions. By breaking the silence and reducing stigma, we can support one another and encourage seeking help when needed.

2. Support Mental Health Organizations: Consider supporting mental health organizations through donations, volunteering, or fundraising activities. These organizations work tirelessly to provide resources, support services, and awareness campaigns. Your contribution, no matter how small, can make a meaningful difference in someone's life.

3. Educate Yourself: Take the initiative to educate yourself further on mental health topics. Read books, articles, and research studies to deepen your understanding of mental health challenges, warning signs, and available resources. This knowledge will enable you to be a supportive ally to those struggling with mental health issues.

4. Practice Self-Care: Prioritize your own mental well-being and practice self-care regularly. Engage in activities that promote relaxation, stress reduction, and emotional well-being, such as exercise, mindfulness, creative outlets, and spending time in nature. Taking care of yourself allows you to be better equipped to support others.

5. Promote Mental Health in your Community: Advocate for mental health initiatives and policies in your community, workplace, or educational institutions. Encourage the implementation of mental health programs, awareness campaigns, and accessible support systems. By championing mental well-being, you can help create a more supportive and inclusive environment for all.

6. Be an Active Listener: Practice active listening when someone shares their experiences or struggles with mental health. Offer empathy, validation, and support without judgment. Sometimes, lending a compassionate ear can provide immense comfort and encouragement to those in need.

7. Engage in Acts of Kindness: Simple acts of kindness can have a positive impact on someone's mental well-being. Extend a helping hand, offer a supportive message, or perform random acts of kindness to brighten someone's day. Small gestures can create a ripple effect of positivity and remind others that they are not alone.

Remember, promoting mental well-being is an ongoing journey. It requires continuous effort, compassion, and understanding. By continuing the conversation, taking action, and fostering a culture of empathy and support, we can create a world where mental health is prioritized, stigma is reduced, and individuals find the help and understanding they deserve.

Let the exploration of Aokigahara Forest be a catalyst for change, inspiring you to make a difference in the lives of those around you and contribute to a more compassionate and mentally healthy society.

Sign up to my free newsletter to get updates on new releases, FREE teaser chapters to upcoming releases and FREE digital short stories.

Or visit https://tinyurl.com/olanc

I never spam and you can unsubscribe at any time.

Don't miss out!

Visit the website below and you can sign up to receive emails whenever Oliver Lancaster publishes a new book. There's no charge and no obligation.

https://books2read.com/r/B-A-UNEZ-LYRLC

BOOKS 2 READ

Connecting independent readers to independent writers.

Also by Oliver Lancaster

Chernobyl: Unveiling the tragedy. A Comprehensive Account of the Nuclear Disaster

The Bhopal Gas Tragedy: Unraveling the Catastrophe of 1984

The Deepwater Horizon Oil Spill of 2010: A Disaster Unveiled

Fukushima Fallout: Unveiling the Truth behind the 2011 Nuclear Disaster

Minamata Disease: Poisoned Waters and the Battle for Justice (1932-1968)

Evil Women: Unmasking History's Most Notorious Women

Bundy The Dark Chronicles: America's Infamous Serial Killer

Dahmer The Dark Chronicles: America's Infamous Milwaukee Cannibal

Zodiac The Dark Chronicles: America's Infamous Cryptic Killer

Bigfoot: The Comprehensive Investigation into the Elusive Legend

Chasing Legends: The Truth behind the Chupacabra

Chasing Legends: The Truth behind the Loch Ness Monster

Aokigahara Forest: The Heartbreaking Secrets of Japan's Suicide Forest

The Amityville House: The Haunting Secrets of America's Most Infamous Residence

The Tower of London: The Haunted Past and Secrets of Royal
Ghosts
The Winchester Mystery House: The Riddle of Sarah
Winchester's Mansion

Watch for more at https://tinyurl.com/olanc.

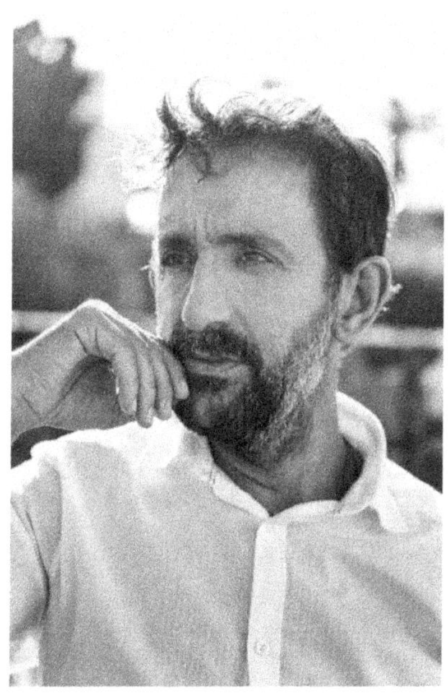

About the Author

Oliver Lancaster possesses an enchanting charm that effortlessly draws readers into the depths of his literary world. With an insatiable curiosity for the unexplained, he skillfully weaves tales of crime, conspiracy, mystery and the unknown, leaving readers on the edge of their seats.

Nestled away in the seclusion of his garden shed, Oliver finds solace and inspiration in the tranquility of nature. Surrounded by greenery and fragrant blooms, he dives into a realm of imagination, unearthing secrets that lie hidden within his mind.

Accompanying Oliver on his literary ventures is his faithful ginger cat named Italics. With his mesmerizing gaze and mysterious mannerisms, Italics adds an air of intrigue to Oliver's writing process, often curling up on a cushioned chair nearby, watching as words flow effortlessly from his human companion's pen.

When not engrossed in his craft, Oliver indulges in the gentle warmth of his garden with a glass of red wine.

Prepare to be spellbound as you delve into the pages of Oliver Lancaster's novels, for he is a master of the eerie, a weaver of secrets, and an unrivaled guide through the labyrinthine corridors of the human psyche.

Sign up to a free newsletter to get updates on new releases, FREE teaser chapters to upcoming releases and FREE digital short stories.

Read more at https://tinyurl.com/olanc.